Psychological Aspects of Surgery

Advances in
Psychosomatic Medicine

Vol. 15

Series Editor
Thomas N. Wise, Falls Church, Va.

Editors
G. Fava, Bologna; *H. Freyberger*, Hannover;
F. Guggenheim, Little Rock, Ark.; *O.W. Hill*, London;
Z.J. Lipowski, Toronto; *G. Lloyd*, Edinburgh;
J.C. Nemiah, Hanover, N.H.; *A. Reading*, Tampa, Fla.;
P. Reich, Boston, Mass.

Consulting Editors
G.L. Engel, Rochester, N.Y.; *H. Weiner*, Bronx, N.Y.;
L. Levi, Stockholm

Editor Emeritus
Franz Reichsmann, Brooklyn, N.Y.

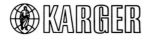 KARGER

Basel · München · Paris · London · New York · New Delhi · Singapore · Tokyo · Sydney

Psychological Aspects of Surgery

Volume Editor
Frederick G. Guggenheim, Little Rock, Ark.

8 figures and 10 tables, 1986

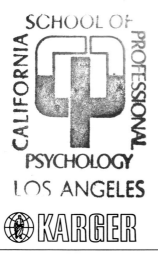

CALIFORNIA SCHOOL OF PROFESSIONAL PSYCHOLOGY

LOS ANGELES

KARGER

Basel · München · Paris · London · New York · New Delhi · Singapore · Tokyo · Sydney

Advances in Psychosomatic Medicine

National Library of Medicine, Cataloging in Publication
Psychological aspects of surgery/
volume editor, Frederick G. Guggenheim.
– Basel; New York: Karger, 1986. –
(Advances in psychosomatic medicine; vol. 15)
Includes index.
1. Surgery, Operative – psychology   I. Guggenheim, Frederick G.   II. Series
Wl AD81 v. 15 [WO 500 P974]
ISBN 3-8055-4090-6

Drug Dosage
The authors and the publisher have exerted every effort to ensure that drug selection and dosage set forth in this text are in accord with current recommendations and practice at the time of publication. However, in view of ongoing research, changes in government regulations, and the constant flow of information relating to drug therapy and drug reactions, the reader is urged to check the package insert for each drug for any change in indications and dosage and for added warnings and precautions. This is particularly important when the recommended agent is a new and/or infrequently employed drug.

Contents

Contributors

Lorraine Dennerstein, MD, Senior Lecturer, Departments of Psychiatry and Obstetrics and Gynecology, University of Melbourne, Melbourne, Australia.

Marshal F. Folstein, MD, Director of General Hospital Psychiatry, Departments of Medicine and Psychiatry and Behavioral Sciences, The Johns Hopkins University School of Medicine, Baltimore, Md.

Gary D. Foster, BA, Department of Psychiatry, University of Pennsylvania School of Medicine, Philadelphia, Pa.

Paul H. Gabriel, MD, Professor of Clinical Psychiatry, Department of Psychiatry, New York University Medical Center; Associate Attending, New York University Hospital and Bellevue Hospital, New York, N.Y.

John M. Goin, MD, Clinical Professor of Surgery, University of Southern California School of Medicine, Los Angeles, Calif.

Marcia K. Goin, MD, PhD, Clinical Professor of Psychiatry, University of Southern California School of Medicine, Los Angeles, Calif.

Richard F. Grossman, BA, Department of Psychiatry, University of Pennsylvania School of Medicine, Philadelphia, Pa.

Frederick G. Guggenheim, MD, Marie Wilson Howells Professor and Chairman, Department of Psychiatry, University of Arkansas for Medical Sciences, Little Rock, Ark.

Stanley Heller, MD, Associate Clinical Professor of Psychiatry College of Physicians and Surgeons at Columbia University; Director, Consultation-Liaison Services, St. Luke Roosevelt Hospital, New York, N.Y.

Jimmie C. Holland, MD, Professor of Psychiatry, Cornell University Medical College; Chief, Psychiatry Service, Memorial Sloan-Kettering Cancer Center, New York, N.Y.

Ellen Jacobs, PhD, Psychology Fellow, Psychiatry Service, Memorial Sloan-Kettering Cancer Center, New York, N.Y.

Marie Johnston, PhD, Senior Lecturer in Clinical Psychology, Royal Free Hospital School of Medicine, University of London, London, England.

Donald Kornfeld, MD, Clinical Professor of Psychiatry, Columbia University, College of Physicians and Surgeons; Chief, Consultation-Liaison Psychiatry Service, Presbyterian Hospital, New York, N.Y.

Norman B. Levy, MD, Professor and Director of Psychiatry, Medicine, and Surgery, New York Medical College; Director, Liaison Psychiatry Division, Westchester County Medical Center, Valhalla, N.Y.

Continuation see page VIII

To Olivia, Hannah and Jennifer Guggenheim

Contributors (Continuation)

Sherry Lundberg, MS, Instructor, Richland College, Dallas, Tex.

Peter Reich, MD, Associate Professor of Psychiatry, Harvard Medical School; Director of Psychiatry, Brigham and Women's Hospital, Boston, Mass.

Malcolm Rogers, MD, Assistant Professor of Psychiatry, Harvard Medical School; Assistant Director, Division of Psychiatry, Brigham and Women's Hospital, Boston, Mass.

Maggie Ryan, BA, MSW, Research Fellow, Departments of Psychiatry and Obstetrics and Gynecology, University of Melbourne, Melbourne, Australia.

Thomas D. Stewart, MD, Assistant Professor of Psychiatry, Harvard Medical School; Director, Consultation-Liaison Service, Beth Israel Hospital, Boston, Mass.

Albert J. Stunkard, MD, Professor of Psychiatry, University of Pennsylvania School of Medicine, Philadelphia, Pa.

Larry Tune, MD, Director, Dementia Research Clinic, Johns Hopkins Hospital, and The Johns Hopkins University School of Medicine, Baltimore, Md.

Adv. psychosom. Med., vol. 15, pp. 1–22 (Karger, Basel 1986)

Pre-Operative Emotional States and Post-Operative Recovery

Marie Johnston

Royal Free Hospital School of Medicine, University of London, London, England

Can we judge from a patient's emotional state prior to surgery how the patient will recover after surgery? The question clearly has important practical clinical implications because an affirmative answer would allow us to identify patients who fare badly with the hope that we might be able to take preventive action. The question also has theoretical implications for the understanding of emotion in more general terms and for the study of environmental stress and how individuals develop methods of coping with stress and risky situations. The interplay between practice and theory is rich. Data from studies of surgical patients have contributed to theories of anxiety and coping which are applied in other clinical spheres such as the treatment of phobic disorders. The theories have produced hypotheses which have been tested on surgical patients and the data have led to new insights relevant to patient care.

In this chapter I seek to answer the initial question both empirically and theoretically. But first some basic clarification of 'pre-operative emotional states' and 'post-operative recovery' is needed.

Pre-Operative Emotional States

By far the most commonly reported and researched pre-operative emotional state is anxiety or fear. Where positive emotions have been measured, they have been negatively correlated with fear-anxiety ratings [1, 2]. Other states such as disgust, hope, boredom, relief, excitement, loneliness and surprise are not usually explored, probably due to their lack of apparent theoretical significance in the study of an event that is seen largely in terms of its stress/threat characteristics. Some important work has been done on depressed/hopeless pre-operative mood in cardiac surgery patients by *Kimball* et al. [3] who showed that such moods were predictive of death in the post-operative period. Moods describing activity level (e.g. energetic, aroused) have also been measured [2, 4].

Despite the possible importance of these other less extensively examined emotions, the main focus of this chapter will be on the pre-operative emotional state variously described as anxiety, fear, stress, etc. This state has been studied in a number of ways, ranging from subjective states, through observable behavioral changes to measures of physiological indices.

The most common approach involves pre-operative assessment of affective state using tests such as the STAI X-1 [5], the MAACL [6] or the POMS [7]. Other measures such as the IPAT, TMAS, STAI X-2 and S-R Inventory assess trait anxiety and are unreliable indices of state anxiety. Various authors including *Spielberger* [5] have drawn attention to the state-trait distinction in anxiety measurement. When considering pre-operative emotion, one is usually referring to the transitory state resulting from the threats associated with the forthcoming surgery and therefore state, rather than the more enduring trait, measures are appropriate. Whether trait measures of anxiety or neuroticism are predictive of high pre-operative state is an empirical question which is considered later in this section.

Using state anxiety measures, it has clearly been demonstrated in a multitude of studies that patients are more anxious prior to surgery than at other times. It is not yet clear how early the anxiety levels rise, consistent elevations having been demonstrated 6 days before surgery, 5 days before admission [8]. Nor is it clear how long the elevated anxiety levels persist; many studies show reduced anxiety after surgery, but the reductions may not occur until some days after surgery rather than immediately [9] and reductions to normal levels may take weeks rather than days [8]. Figure 1 demonstrates the affective state, measured by the STAI pre- and post-operatively for 72 patients [8].

Other studies have measured situation specific anxiety, asking patients to rate how worried or concerned they feel about: being in the hospital, the prospect of surgery and the prospect of anesthesia [2, 10–13]. These measures produce similar results to the state anxiety measures taken pre-operatively.

An alternative approach has been to examine cognitive content, exploring what patients think or worry about throughout the period in the hospital for surgery [14–19]. Surgical patients, compared to medical patients, are

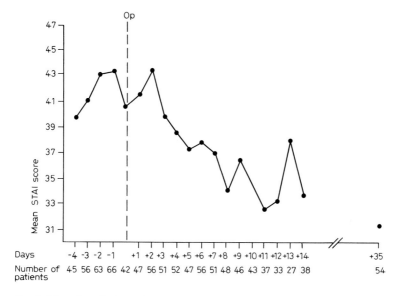

Fig. 1. Mean State Trait Anxiety Inventory (STAI) scores daily for total sample of 72 patients.

more troubled by the unfamiliarity of surroundings, loss of independence and threat of severe illness [20]. These studies also demonstrate that the worries and concerns of surgical patients are not confined to the threatening elements of the hospital situation. For example, home and family worries are amongst the most commonly cited and most severe worries [16, 18, 19, 21]. Thus pre-operative worries also include worries external to the immediate situation in addition to worries about anesthesia and surgery.

When anxiety has been measured by observers' ratings, the results have followed the patient's self-report measures of affective state or amount of anxiety [1, 18, 22]. It would appear that the patient's *level* of anxiety is revealed to these observers, either indirectly or by direct communication, in a reliable manner. However nurse observers seem unable to describe the cognitive *content* of the patient's worries [18, 19]. Thus observers may be more able to detect that a patient is anxious than to know what they are anxious about. *Baer* et al. [23] present analogue studies which suggest that distress is communicated by verbal rather than non-verbal behavior and therefore it is surprising that the content should not be connected with the degree of anxiety.

More complex measurement of pre-operative emotion has involved physiological recording. *Harrison* et al. [24] and *Johnson* et al. [2] have used measures of palmar sweating. *Williams* [25] have developed a skin conductance anxiety test, with anxiety being indexed by the dosage of sodium Thiopental required to cause stabilization of spontaneous GSR's. This latter measure was found to correlate with IPAT scores and may therefore reflect trait anxiety. While palmar sweating is correlated with subjective reports of stress or anxiety in many settings, this is not true for surgical patients. The earliest study [24] found that palmar sweating declined as surgery approached, reaching a minimum on the day following surgery, with subsequent increases to normal levels taking an average of 10 days to 2 weeks. Thus rather than following the time course of anxiety changes, the palmar sweating measure shows an opposite pattern. The results are not due to pre-operative medication, nor the changes occurring prior to such medication, nor are they due to hospitalization for medical patients do not show such changes. The pattern of results has been replicated in two studies [26, 27] where subjective anxiety/fear was also measured; palmar sweating appeared to be unrelated to subjective anxiety. *Johnson* et al. [26] found that the mood most closely related to palmar sweating changes in surgical patients was lethargy. They suggest that this may reflect the shift in attention from the external to the internal environment, with a later shift to the external environment in the post-surgical phases.

Other physiological indices of stress have shown changes prior to surgery and prior to the effects of pre-medication anesthesia. *Burnstein and Ross* [28] found a positive relationship between plasma corticosteroid levels and pre-operative trait anxiety (TMAS). *Fleishman* et al. [29] found relationships between pre-operative STAI X-1 (state anxiety) and blood pressure, heart rate and platelet aggregation time, but only limited evidence of a relationship with corticosteroid levels. *Sane and Kukreti* [30] found raised serum cholesterol levels in patients of all age groups both before and after surgery, the initial effects being detected on admission to the hospital with further rises before surgery. *Corenblum and Taylor* [31] attempted to separate the effects of apprehension about surgery and the direct effects of anesthesia/surgery stress in studies of prolactin levels. They found evidence that both stressors increased prolactin levels but that the increases were probably achieved by different mechanisms, apprehension leading to release of prolactin-releasing factor, anesthesia/surgery to inhibition of prolactin-inhibiting factor. With the exception of Corenblum and Taylor's study, these studies do little to clarify the nature of the physiological response to stress involved in pre-surgical anxiety.

Thus while the data on subjective anxiety and observer rated anxiety presents a coherent picture, and there is some agreement on the nature of pre-operative cognitions, the relationship between levels of subjective anxiety and physiological measures is not at all clear.

In choosing a measure of pre-operative emotion, it is important to choose one that is consistent with the theory or practice being explored, as it is impossible to extrapolate from one to another. Thus palmar sweating will give no index of subjective anxiety, and raters' assessments of patients' worries are unlikely to match self-reported worries.

With these caveats about the measurement of pre-operative emotion, it is possible to turn briefly to predictors of pre-operative anxiety.

The most obvious predictor is trait anxiety [8, 13, 32]; it has consistently been shown that those who are most anxious prior to surgery are anxious people generally. There are sex differences in that women report more anxieties than men [33, 34].

Post-Operative Recovery

Recovery from surgery has been measured by length of stay, ambulation on the ward, emotional distress, pain, medication, post-operative complications, blood pressure, heart rate, return to normal activities, return to work, death, etc. It is doubtful whether all of these indices are measuring the same thing or even if the authors have the same concept of recovery. Sometimes there is confusion between recovery from the disease or illness and recovery from the procedure. On other occasions there is confusion between what the patient can do and what the individual surgeon will allow or encourage. Many studies have failed to find correlations between different measures of recovery [1, 2, 22, 35, 36].

This chapter takes a liberal view of recovery measurement, including whatever the authors thought relevant. Elsewhere I have argued that these measures not only fail to measure the same dimension, but some may not even reflect improvements in the patient's state [36]. However even liberal overinclusiveness requires organization.

The results of a principal component analysis of post-operative outcome measures suggests a possible organization, as presented in table I. The analysis demonstrated stable and replicable components of Recovery and Distress (also called well-being and emotional distress) with a further less reliable Pain component. These three components include many of the measures used to assess recovery. A further component, dealing with patients' attitudes to care, is not relevant in the current context. Thus a three-fold classification of post-operative variables is suggested.

Two amendments to the principal component classification have been adopted. Measures of length of stay and post-operative complications have been tabulated with *Recovery* although they were not included in the original analysis. Secondly, use of drugs, particularly sedatives and analgesics, did not load consistently on any component, but is a common outcome measure; it has been considered separately to give a four-fold classification (Recovery, Distress, Pain and Drugs). These four plus an unclassified 'other' section in the table organize information about post-operative recovery.

Relationships between Pre-Operative and Post-Operative States

Table I summarizes the main studies relating pre-operative emotional states and post-operative measures. Studies of children and dental patients have been excluded as they are in many ways different from studies of typical adult surgical patients. Studies of children are more likely to focus on long term post-discharge effects and dental surgery is often confounded with the stress associated with normal, non-surgical dental procedures. The pre-operative measures include measures of transient states, moods and coping styles, but exclude more enduring trait measures. The post-operative measures have been separated into the five categories discussed above.

It is clear that, where pre-operative anxiety, fear of surgery, depression and stress have been measured, they relate positively to post-operative distress (9 significant findings). The only exception is the original *Janis* work [37] where a curvilinear relationship was found, moderate pre-operative anxiety leading to minimal post-operative distress. Other studies which have systematically explored this relationship have supported a linear relationship and have found no evidence of increased post-operative distress in patients with low pre-operative anxiety [see reference 12].

Self-report anxiety and stress measures are also related, although not so clearly, to post-operative pain (4 positive and 1 negative relationship significant, 3 non-significant). Only one anxiety measure is related to post-operative drug consumption, which would appear to be more closely related to cop-

Table I. Studies relating pre-operative and post-operative states

Authors	Pre-operative state	Post-operative state					Surgery
		distress	pain	drugs	recovery	other	
Janis 1958	anxiety	C					mixed
Wolfer and Davis 1970	fear/anxiety	+					gynaecology, major abdominal
Johnson et al. 1971	fear	+	+	n.s.	n.s.		hysterectomy, cholecystectomy
	fear of surgery	+	+	n.s.	n.s.		
Cohen and Lazarus 1973	anxiety	+	n.s.	n.s.	n.s.		mixed
	vigilance	n.s.	n.s.	n.s.	−		
	observed		n.s.	n.s.	n.s.		
	anxiety	n.s.					
Auerbach 1973	anxiety	+					mixed
	anxiety elevation	n.s.				attitudes C	
Martinez-Urrutia 1975	fear of surgery		−				mixed
Sime 1976	fear of surgery	+		+	−		abdominal
	information seeking	n.s.		n.s.	n.s.		
Chapman and Cox 1977	depression	+					abdominal
Volicer 1978	hospital stress		+		−		mixed
Johnston and Carpenter 1980	anxiety	+	n.s.		n.s.		major gynaecology
	fear of surgery	+	n.s.		n.s.		
Wilson 1981	fear of surgery				−	epinephrine +	cholecystectomy/ hysterectomy
	denial			−	+		
	aggressiveness			+	−		
Ray and Fitzgibbon 1981	stress	+	+	n.s.	n.s.		cholecystectomy
	arousal	n.s.	−	−	+		

+ = Positive relationship; − = negative relationship; C = curvilinear relationship; n.s. = non-significant relationship.

ing style; denial and arousal are both negatively related to post-operative medication.

Finally, indices of recovery suggest that the process may be slower and more complicated in patients with high levels of pre-operative anxiety/stress, this relationship being significant in 3 out of the 10 reported assessments. Coping strategy measures suggest faster recovery with avoidance rather than vigilance, with denial, and with more active, aroused pre-operative styles.

In practical, clinical terms it would appear that high pre-operative fear or anxiety is predictive of poor post-operative outcomes of all kinds. Thus the more fearful pre-operative patient is later likely to be more emotionally upset, to experience more pain and perhaps require more medication and to have a slower recovery than the patient who is less anxious about surgery. There is no reason to believe that a modicum of anxiety is useful as originally proposed by *Janis* [37] since subsequent studies have failed to find evidence of a beneficial effect of anxiety. Therefore, on this basis, one can conclude that reducing patients pre-operative anxiety should improve post-operative outcomes without any risk of harm to the patient with lower anxiety. Further evidence comes from studies which attempt to lower patients' anxiety and change their coping strategies (intervention studies and their outcomes are discussed in the following chapter).

Explanations of the Relationship between Pre-Operative Emotional and Cognitive States and Post-Operative States

The possible theoretical significance of the findings relating pre- and post-operative states is discussed in the context of the current explanatory theories. A number of hypotheses allow prediction of the patient's post-operative state from the pre-operative emotional and cognitive state. Eight current theories that have important implications for the care of surgical patients are discussed here.

Emotional Drive

The best known and most influential theory derives from *Janis's* [37] work. He proposed: that anxiety serves a useful pre-operative function as it causes patients to engage in preparatory mental activity, 'the work of worrying'; and that the quality and quantity of this worry determines the post-operative emotional state. If patients experienced too little anxiety, they would fail to do the work of worrying and would therefore be unprepared for the pain, discomfort, and restrictions of the post-operative period; their subsequent experience might lead to distress with the possibility of irritability and anger expressed towards nurses and other staff. *Janis* also considered the patients with high anxiety to be at risk; but they were at risk because their worry might include a wide range of worries unrelated to the immediate surgical threat with the result that they too would be unprepared for the post-operative period. Thus *Janis* predicted that a moderate amount of pre-operative anxiety leads to the optimal pre-operative mental preparation and resulting post-operative emotional state.

From a clinical rather than theoretical point of view, this theory had important practical implications: it allowed two groups of patients at risk of high post-operative distress to be identified pre-operatively with the possibility that one might intervene to reduce this risk. *Janis* suggested that for both groups, giving pre-operative information about the impending surgery should be beneficial, for the low-anxious group by increasing their anxiety levels and thus inducing the work of worrying, and for the high anxious group by identifying the range of appropriate worries.

Janis' research with surgical patients supported his hypothesized U-shaped relationship between pre- and post-operative anxiety and distress. But subsequent studies have been critical of *Janis'* methodology and have found results which support a linear relationship [see 12]. Indeed evidence of *Janis'* U-shaped relationship is minimal. *Auerbach* [38] did find a U-shaped relationship between pre-operative anxiety elevation and post-operative attitudes to hospital care. He studied the increase in patients' anxiety prior to surgery rather than simply the level of pre-operative anxiety and found that those patients who had moderate increases in anxiety before surgery had the most favorable attitudes. While the critical attitudes of patients with small anxiety elevation may be consistent with the prediction of irritability and anger in the post-operative period, other studies which have looked more directly for evidence of this post-operative mood have found it unrelated to low pre-operative anxiety [12, 26]. A reverse of the expected U-curve, i.e. showing moderate pre-operative anxiety to predict the poorest post-operative outcome, was found with one recovery measure by *Johnston* [21] and with length of hospitalization in *Sime's* [10] group of well-informed patients.

These results appear to thoroughly refute the original emotional drive theory but the alternative approaches almost all owe something if not to the original theory, at least to the findings of the research spawned by the theory.

Parallel Response

Leventhal [39] introduced the parallel-response model as an alternative to the emotional drive model. Based on work outside the field of surgery, the model proposes that there are 2 independent responses to a threatening stimulus: attempts to deal with fear and attempts to deal with and possibly avert impending danger. The fear response does not cause danger control. Rather these two responses occur in parallel, e.g., in the surgical situation, it is not the pre-surgical experience of fear that causes the patient to prepare to control pain. The recognition of threats also causes fear, but this process is independent. Thus, pre-operative fear should not be predictive of post-operative danger control.

Johnson et al. [2] found support for this model in a study which showed that emotionality measures did not predict indices of danger control. Instead, danger control was predictable from locus of control measures indicating the extent to which the individual felt able to control what happened. Measures of pre-operative emotional distress were linearly related to post-operative distress and the authors interpreted this finding as being consistent with the parallel response model. However, although the linear relationship is consistent with the model, it is hardly predicted. The model deals with fear elicited on discrete occasions, and fear on one occasion does not predict fear on a future occasion. If danger control were effective (e.g. in soliciting adequate analgesia and thereby reducing pain) one might expect less post-operative fear as the danger had been reduced. But this danger control is quite independent of pre-operative fear. Therefore there is no clear reason for the model to predict a relationship, linear or otherwise, between pre- and post-operative fear.

This approach usefully separates two components of the pre-operative state, the emotion/fear control component and the instrumental/danger control component. Whereas *Janis* suggested that pre-operative communications could usefully increase the anxiety of the low anxious pre-operative patient, *Leventhal's* model suggests that increasing anxiety would serve no function and that one might either aim to reduce pre-operative anxiety simply to reduce discomfort, or one might aim to give information leading to more effective danger control post-operatively with possible reductions in distress after surgery. These ideas are developed in other models.

Predictability

A wide range of human and animal literature [40] demonstrates that predictable events cause less emotional response than the unpredictable. Surgical patients are often described as experiencing 'fear of the unknown'. One might argue that surgical patients who are unable to predict what will happen after surgery should experience more distress than those for whom the event is predictable. In surgical patients, information about procedures is frequently given with the aim of increasing predictability and reducing distress. *Johnson* [41] has suggested that in order to reduce distress, it is most important to be able to predict sensations associated with threatening stimuli. In a series of studies giving patients information about sensations or information about procedures, her hypothesis about the superiority of sensation information tended to be supported [42–45]. However other evidence suggests that increasing predictability does not necessarily reduce post-operative distress.

Staite [46] compared a preparatory communication group given information about sensations which would be experienced, with a control communication group in a study of patients having major gynecological surgery. There was no difference between the two groups of subjects on any of the post-operative measures of mood, pain, recovery, or length of stay. However, the groups did differ on their post-operative ratings of the accuracy of their expectations: the informed or preparatory group described their expectations as more accurate than did the control group. Clearly it was possible to increase predictability without reducing distress. A number of studies have now been completed in which pre-operative information, which presumably increased predictability of events, did not lead to reduced distress. Indeed *Visser* [13] found that patients given a pre-operative information booklet showed higher post-operative anxiety than those given no booklet, although he suggests that this may be due to confounding sample characteristics.

Accuracy of expectations can also be examined by asking patients to predict pre-operatively and then compare the prediction with the reported post-operative experience. *Johnston* [47] asked patients to predict post-operative pain, measured actual post-operative pain and calculated the absolute inaccuracy of prediction i.e. the difference between expected and actual pain scores irrespective of direction of difference. There was no relationship between this calculated score and the amount of emotional distress reported by patients post-operatively. Instead, emotional distress was associated with underestimates of expected pain i.e., having more pain than anticipated whether the patient estimated a low amount or a high amount. This result was not simply attributable to patients with higher post-operative pain: giving low estimates of expected pain was also predictive of greater post-operative distress. Nor was it due to the more emotional patients giving low estimates of pain: there was no relationship between expected pain values and concurrent anxiety scores.

These results suggest that predictability is not the main determinant of distress as *Johnson* would assert. Rather more important is that the anticipation should encompass the actual experience. The patient can better afford to have a wildly inaccurate but overestimated expectation of pain than a midly inaccurate but underestimated expectation of pain. One might hypothesize that patients prepare themselves for the amount of pain that they anticipate. This notion has some appeal, being consistent with the danger control aspects of the parallel response model and even with those aspects of *Janis'* model which suggest that mental pre-operative preparation may be useful. However, it also suggests that it is important that the anticipated danger should not be underestimated and that pre-operative communications may fail if they go too far in reducing the patient's estimate of risks. Unlike *Janis'* hypothesis which considers that anxiety levels may be too low, this hypothesis envisages the possibility of an estimation of danger that is too low, leading to inadequate preparation and inability to control the danger.

Controllability

The above discussion suggests that patients may cope well post-operatively when events are within their capacity to control. Evidence from human and animal studies predominately [40] indicates reduced emotional responses where the subjects perceive that they can control the danger stimulus, even when this perception is false. *Leventhal's* parallel response model suggests that fearfulness should be reduced when the danger has been controlled and the threat no longer exists.

In the surgical situation, there are limits to the amount of danger control the patient can exercise, as most dangers are controlled by medical and nursing staff. When investigations have measured control, they have used indices that reflect the patient's influence over nursing and medical decisions such as 'success in obtaining pain-relieving medications' [2] or increased days of hospitalization. These measures, which are taken to indicate increases in danger control in some studies, are used in other studies to indicate poor recovery, and therefore the same measure may indicate a good or a poor outcome. Intervention studies often try to introduce behaviors which will reduce the potency of noxious stimuli e.g. by teaching patients to relax the area of incision, or how to cough or move, or how to use apparatus available to the patient, all of which would appear to introduce an element of danger control. Alternatively the intervention may introduce fear control either by a muscle relaxation procedure or by a cognitive strategy. Psychological interventions are discussed in the following chapter and will not be elaborated here. However each intervention has importance not only as method of improving clinical outcomes but also as a test of theoretical models of how patients cope with surgery. The evidence would suggest that when patients are trained in methods of controlling either fear or danger, there are likely to be improvements in post-operative states.

Control may also be considered in terms of the patients' personal style rather than as a feature of the environment or a specific adaptive skill. If perceived control is helpful in reducing stress, then patients who perceive themselves to have more control should fare better than others, regardless of whether they have more control. A number of studies have used locus of control measured by *Rotter's* I-E scale and found rather mixed results [2, 48]. It might be more appropriate to examine situation-specific measures of control, i.e., how the individual tries to control events in the surgical situation. The data in table I referring to vigilance and denial suggest that a style which surrenders control is more adaptive than a controlling style. Thus the patient's style may determine the optimal level of control.

Personality Style

In addition to locus of control, various other persistent characteristics of the patients, considered either as personality features or dominant coping styles, have been explored as possible predictors of post-operative state. The most obvious and simple predictors are measures of trait anxiety. In order to identify patients who will be most distressed and anxious in the post-operative period, one would gain greatest success by administering a test of trait anxiety. This has been illustrated in many studies [2, 32]. In addition, *Johnston* [47] has further examined the linear relationship between pre- and post-operative anxiety controlling for trait anxiety levels using the State-Trait Anxiety Inventory [5]. The results showed that the linear relationship disappeared when the effects of trait anxiety were removed. The most appropriate explanation of the linear relationship, the most consistent finding in table I, is therefore a personality or a temperament explanation, e.g., anxious people tend to get anxious in anxiety provoking situations including pre- and post-operative situations. As such the results may reveal little about coping with surgery except that high and low anxious people cope differently.

Alternatively, the critical personality style may be willingness to report distress, producing a similar bias in reporting pre- and post-operatively. This possibility is considered in section 7 on communication hypotheses. *Mathews and Ridgeway* [49] conclude that anxiety or neuroticism measures of personality are the most clearly demonstrated predictors of post-operative states, but they also suggest that other variables which have intermittent predictive success do so because they are correlated with trait anxiety. For example, measures of repression-sensitization and avoidance-vigilance have been shown to correlate with EPI neuroticism or other trait anxiety measures. However, these other measures may offer some insights into the cognitive style of the anxious person.

Cognitive Hypotheses

Many of the hypotheses considered so far are partly cognitive. If the emotional drive aspect of *Janis's* hypothesis is ignored, then the remainder of the theory says that the content of the patient's thoughts in the pre-operative period i.e., the extent to which they reflect on the forthcoming operation, will determine subsequent performance. Both the perceived controllability model and the appraisal of threat in the parallel response model contain cognitive parameters. Moreover, many of the approaches to personality style involve an identified cognitive component.

Cognitive hypotheses attribute a causal role to the thoughts of the patient in determining outcomes. The simplest versions assert that the patient's self-talk i.e., what the patient says to him or her self, affects outcomes [50, 51].

Many authors have considered that patients may be at risk of post-operative distress if they do not think about the operation in advance. This cognitive style may be considered either as a defense mechanism or as a coping strategy. For example, *Janis* considers that the defense mechanisms of denial, leading both to low reported anxiety levels and to low awareness of threats associated with surgery, leaves the patient vulnerable in the post-operative period when these defences can no longer be maintained as the patient actually experiences pain. The fact that subsequent research has been unable to identify a group of low anxiety patients who are particularly at risk [12] suggests that this hypothesis is either untenable or at least has not been specified in enough detail to be tested or applied. The coping strategy approach suggests that patients adopt a style of thinking about the operation, either a habitual style of coping with stress or one elicited by this particular stress.

Two sets of studies examine the issue of avoiding thinking about the forthcoming procedure as a coping device. *Wilson* [35] found that patients who described themselves as coping with stress by using high levels of denial actually had shorter hospital stays and consumed fewer analgesic medications than patients who described themselves as low deniers. Somewhat in concert, *Cohen and Lazarus* [22] identified patients as adopting avoidant or vigilant coping strategies, the vigilant patients attending more to information about their medical condition and surgery. They found that the best post-operative outcomes were associated with the avoidant style. This result might lead one to question the evaluative nature of the labels 'avoidant' and 'vigilant'. In so far as their measures indicate the amount of thought the patient gives to the future operation, the results contradict a notion that actively thinking about the operation is useful in promoting recovery. *Cohen and Lazarus* [22, 52] suggest that the vigilant patient attempts to master the situation and that this is maladaptive post-operatively as there is nothing that can be actively mastered. Also, the vigilant patient may be attempting to master many threats, few of which actually materialize. This latter explanation brings the vigilant patient closer to *Janis's* idea of the high anxiety patient, whose work of worrying is not sufficiently focused to be adaptive. *Mathew and Ridgeway* [49] suggest that vigilance is more akin to anxiety in which case the results would be consistent with other findings.

Thus the evidence does not support the hypotheses that actively thinking about the operation is useful, and this may be because the amount of time spent thinking about the operation is related to neuroticism. Measures such as denial or avoidance-vigilance appear to describe quantity rather than quality of thoughts and actually the latter may be the key variable. Thus a number of successful cognitive interventions have encouraged patients to think about the operation in a particular way involving positive interpretations, rather than altering the amount of time spent thinking [50, 53]. *Ray* [54] suggests that surgical patients must not only cope with their emotions and the danger of surgery, but also with the meaning of the situation, the extent to which it is viewed optimistically or pessimistically and so on.

There is evidence that patients with higher anxiety levels may have a different quality as well as quantity of thoughts about the operation. *Johnston* [21] found that the main worries of pre-operative patients with high anxiety levels were more likely to be idiosyncratic and not shared by other patients having similar surgery than those of patients with low anxiety. All of the patients with low anxiety shared at least one of the common worries of the group. This result, in conjunction with the results of the cognitive intervention studies, allows the possibility that certain thoughts or types of thought may be more adaptive and that a cognitive hypothesis remains tenable.

Communication Hypotheses

It is widely accepted that communication with the patient, whether specifically designed for the purpose or as part of normal spontaneous social interaction, may affect post-operative outcomes. The patient's pre-operative state may influence these communications and so influence post-operative measures indirectly by changing the type of reassurance given or by biasing staff's thinking about the extent of clinical progress.

Firstly, certain forms of communication may be inappropriate, given certain personality styles and emotional states of the patient. For example, attempts to reassure a patient are likely to be effective to the extent that the reassurance is compatible with the patient's style and concerns. *Miller* [55] found pre-operative communications were most effective when they took account of 'monitoring'/'blocking', the patient's preference for attending to/or ignoring the threatening situation.

Subgroups of patients have been identified who have worse outcomes as a result of pre-operative communications. One can argue that this was due to incompatibility between the communication and the patient's response style [56]. For example *Andrew* [57] found that avoiders required increased pain medication when given preparatory communications. *Sime* [10] found that patients with moderate pre-operative fear who reported receiving much information had longer post-operative hospital stays than those who received little information.

Evidence suggests that nurses are very inaccurate in assessing patients' worries and are likely to be accurate, and therefore have the opportunity for appropriate reassurance, only with the patients who have the more common worries [18, 19]. As suggested above, patients with common worries may be those with low anxiety. Therefore better outcomes found in low anxious patients may be achieved because such patients have been adequately reassured about their worries. The same research also showed that patients know more about each other's worries than the nurses do, and so other patients might serve as an alternative source of reassurance for the low anxious patients. However, they too are likely to be best equipped to reassure about common worries and additionally, are less likely to be seen as an appropriate source of support [58].

Quite a different kind of communication hypothesis concerns the degree to which communications from the patient to their caregivers affect the outcome indices and bias care. If patients are unwilling to report distress, then they may not only show low levels of anxiety before and after surgery in response to research interventions and questions, but also report less post-operative distress to hospital staff who in turn respond by reducing medication and promoting an early discharge from the hospital. This would certainly fit the data supporting the linear relationship between pre- and post-operative distress and the evidence of good outcomes for avoiders and deniers. These two hypotheses, about access to reassurance and reporting bias, are relatively untested.

Physiological Hypotheses
Anxiety/Anesthesia

Williams [59] has proposed that patients with high pre-operative anxiety require more anaesthetic to achieve adequate levels of sedation and are therefore slower to recover post-operatively. This hypothesis would offer a possible explanation of the relationship between pre-operative anxiety and post-operative recovery, but the evidence *Williams* reports is based on a physiological index of anxiety. Since others have shown that related skin conductance measures do not relate to subjective anxiety in surgical patients [26], this relationship may be spurious.

Stress/Immunity

Bradley [60] suggests that psychological stress associated with surgery may, by increasing secretion of ACTH and thus corticosteroids, inhibit the immune response and therefore depress resistance to infection, resulting in a slower recovery. This important hypothesis receives indirect support from studies of stresses other than surgery. Additionally, in an intervention study of surgical patients given a complex pre-operative information package, *Boore* [61] showed that the control group had higher levels of 17-hydroxycorticosteroid and a greater incidence of post-operative infections than the informed group. Also *Kinney* [62] found that pre-operative instructions were associated with higher circulating lymphocyte counts than in the control group in patients preparing for cardiac surgery. These psychological interventions are consistent with *Bradley's* hypothesis that psychological as well as anesthetic and other physical stresses are involved. *Corenblum and Taylor* [31] have found evidence that both apprehension about surgery and the effect of anesthesia/surgery lead to elevated serum prolactin levels in surgical patients.

This hypothesis offers a further possible mediating mechanism for the relationship between pre-operative anxiety and recovery from surgery. It may also be capable of explaining the effects of cognitive style, as there is some evidence that avoidant copers have reduced secretion of corticosteroids. Those parents of children with leukemia who used a denial coping approach had lower urinary corticosteroids than other parents [63].

Conclusions

Despite the complexity of the pre-operative measures and the diversity of the post-operative parameters, it is possible to conclude that high pre-operative anxiety leads to poor post-operative outcomes and that low pre-operative anxiety leads to good outcomes. There may be certain predisposing characteristics of the individual, especially trait anxiety, that determine the degree of pre-operative anxiety reached. These features may be useful in identifying patients at risk for problems after surgery.

There are many models relating pre-operative anxiety and post-operative outcomes. At one extreme is a psycho-physiological explanation, with experienced anxiety triggering a neuro-endocrine chain pre-operatively which then has a deleterious effect on the post-operative recovery pattern. At the other extreme is a behavioral-communication explanation in which the patient's disclosure of distress influences both the pre-operative measures of anxiety and also the post-operative assessment and responses of nursing and medical staff regarding the patient's physical state. Between these two extremes lie the more popular explanations with cognitive-behavioral and physiological explanations running in parallel. In each case, the patient's thoughts in the pre-operative period are considered important in determining the adequacy of post-operative coping. Before and after surgery, appraisal of the situation as being beyond the individual's capacity to cope leads both to anxiety and to associated physiological stress responses in the pituitary adreno-cortical axis. Changes in the adreno-medullary axis may reflect the active coping adopted by the patient.

These explanations have important but varying implications for patient management and for understanding stress mechanisms. It is obviously essential to establish whether relationships between pre-operative and post-operative states are mediated by changes in physical functioning. Very few studies have measured both physiological and psychological parameters. Repeated measures of patients before and after surgery could clarify these issues.

A second area which requires further research is ward communication including both the normal procedures for reassuring and preparing patients, and also the role of communications between patients. The possibility that the patient's communications style may influence post-operative care by altering staff perceptions of their level of recovery is also worth investigating.

A considerable amount of work is currently being done on cognitive coping styles. It seems likely that these will offer better predictions of post-operative recovery than measure of the pre-operative emotional state. However this work is difficult to assimilate because of varying measures of coping style and the lack of testable and tested hypotheses about the mechanisms involved. It is unlikely that further work on coping will advance the field unless the possible causal pathways are explored at the same time. It will also be necessary to have clear definitions of both pre-operative coping and post-operative recovery variables. Since the usual indices of recovery do not all measure the same dimension, it may be possible to find that some styles of coping benefit certain types of recovery but not others while alternative coping styles are effective in other ways.

In an area where beliefs are inclined to swamp the evidence, it may be worthwhile to summarize the practical implications of the research reviewed.

---

1) Highly anxious patients are likely to be highly anxious after surgery and may have a slower recovery.

2) Low anxious patients are likely to do well post-operatively.

3) Clinical staff may be able to identify anxious patients without understanding what they are anxious about.

4) Patients who avoid opportunities to learn about their operation are not necessarily at risk post-surgically, and may do well.

5) Having inaccurate expectations about surgery is more likely to lead to problems post-operatively if the difficulties are underestimated.

6) Patients may attempt to control either their emotions or the actual threats of surgery.

7) Patients are more likely to be highly anxious if they are young, female or neurotic, have an excess of recent life events, or are suffering from a more stressful medical condition.

8) Patients displaying an active, energetic mood pre-operatively are likely to demonstrate fast post-operative recovery.

9) Neuro-endocrine disturbance is associated both with the anticipation of surgery and with the actual procedures.

10) Palmar sweating and experienced anxiety levels do not change together over time in surgical patients.

References

1   Wolfer, J.; Davis, C.E.: Assessment of surgical patients pre-operative emotional condition and post-operative welfare. Nursing Research *19:* 402–414 (1970).

2   Johnson, J.; Leventhal, H.; Dabbs, J.M.: Contribution of emotional and instrumental response processes in adaptation to surgery. J. Pers. Soc. Psychol. *20:* 55–64 (1971).

3   Kimball, C.P.: Psychological responses to the experience of open heart surgery. I. Am. J. Psychiat. *126:* 96–107 (1969).

4   Ray, C.; Fitzgibbon, G.: Stress arousal and coping with surgery. Psychol. Med. *11:* 741–746 (1981).

5   Spielberger, C.D.; Gorsuch, R.L.; Lushene, R.E.: State Trait Anxiety Inventory Manual. Consult. Psychol. Press, Palo Alto (1970).

6   Zuckerman, M.; Lubin, B.: Multiple affect adjective check list manual (Educational and Industrial Testing Service, San Diego, 1965).

7   Lorr, M.; Daston, P.; Smith, I.R.: An analysis of mood states. Educational and Psychological Measurement *27:* 89–96 (1967).

8   Johnston, M.: Anxiety in surgical patients. Psychol. Med. *10:* 145–152 (1980).

9   Chapman, C.R.; Cox, G.B.: Determinants of anxiety in dental surgery patients; in Spielberger and Sarason, Stress and Anxiety *4,* pp. 269–290 (Wiley, New York, 1977).

10 Sime, M.: Relationship of pre-operative fear, type of coping, and information received about surgery to recovery from surgery. J. Pers. Soc. Psychol. *34:* 716–724 (1976).

11 Martinez-Urrutia, A.: Anxiety and pain in surgical patients. J. Consult. Clin. Psychol. *43:* 437–442 (1975).

12 Johnston, M.; Carpenter, L.: Relationship between pre-operative anxiety and post-operative state. Psychol. Med. *10:* 361–367 (1980).

13 Visser, A.: Situational and individual determinants of state anxiety of surgical patients; in Spielberger, Defares and Sarason, Stress and Anxiety (Academic, New York, 1982).

14 Lucente, F.E.; Fleck, S.: A study of hospitalization anxiety in 408 medical and surgical patients. Psychosom. Med. *34:* 304–312 (1972).

15 DeWolfe, A.S.; Barrell, R.P.; Cummings, J.W.: Patient variables in emotional response to hospitalization for physical illness. J. Consult. Clin. Psychol. *30:* 68–72 (1966).

16 Volicer, B.J.; Bohannon, M.W.: A hospital stress rating scale. Nursing Research *24:* 352–359 (1975).

17 Wilson-Barnett, J.: Patients' emotional reactions to hospitalization: an explanatory study. J. Adv. Nursing *1:* 351–358 (1976).

18 Johnston, M.: Communication of patients' feelings in hospital; in Bennett, M., Communication Between Doctors and Patients, pp. 30–43 (Oxford University Press, Oxford, 1976).

19 Johnston, M.: Recognition of patients worries by nurses and by other patients. Br. J. Clin. Psychol. *21:* 255–261 (1982).

20 Volicer, B.J.; Isenberg, M.A.; Burns, M.W.: Medical-Surgical differences in hospital stress factors. J. Hum. Stress *3:* 3–13 (1977).

21 Johnston, M.: Anxiety and worries in surgical patients; in Van der Ploeg and Defares, Stress en Angst in de Medische Situatie, pp. 131–143 (Stafleu, Alphen aan den Rijn, 1982).

22 Cohen, F.; Lazarus, R.S.: Active coping processes, coping dispositions, and recovery from surgery. Psychosom. Med. *35:* 375–389 (1973).

23 Baer, E.; Davitz, L.J.; Lieb, R.: Interferences of physical pain in relation to verbal and non-verbal patient communication. Nursing Research *5:* 388–391 (1970).

24 Harrison, J.; MacKinnon, P.; Monk-Jones, M.E.: Behavior of the palmar sweat glands before and after operation. Clin. Sci. *23:* 371–377 (1962).

25 Williams, J.G.L.; Jones, J.R.; Williams, B.: A physiological measure of pre-operative anxiety. Psychosom. Med. *41:* 522–527 (1969).

26 Johnson, J.E.; Dabbs, J.M.; Leventhal, H.: Psychosocial factors in the welfare of surgical patients. Nursing Research 19: 18–28 (1970).

27 Johnston, M.: Stress and Surgery. (Paper presented at the British Psychological Society Conference, December 1982). Conference Proceedings: Abstract in Bulletin of the British Psychological Society 36: A8–A9 (1983).

28 Burnstein, B.; Russ, J.J.: Pre-operative psychological state and corticosteroid levels of surgical patients. Psychosom. Med. 27: 309–317 (1965).

29 Fleishman, A.I.; Bierenbaum, M.; Stier, A.: Effect of stress due to anticipated minor surgery upon in vivo platelet aggregation in humans. J. Hum. Stress 2: 33–37 (1976).

30 Sane, A.S.; Kukreti, S.C.: Effect of pre-operative stress on serum cholesterol level in humans. Experementia 34: 213–244 (1978).

31 Corenblum, B.; Taylor, J.: Mechanisms of control of prolactin release in response to apprehension stress and anaesthesia/surgery stress. Fert. Steril. 36: 712–715 (1981).

32 Spielberger, C.D.; Auerbach, S.M.; Wadsworth, A.P.; Dunn, T.M.; Taulbee, E.S.: Emotional reactions to surgery. J. Consult. Clin. Psychol. 40: 33–38 (1973).

33 French, K.: Some anxieties of elective surgery patients and the desire for reassurance and information; in Oborne, Gruneberg and Eiser, Research in Psychology and Medicine, No. 2, pp. 336–343 (Academic, London, 1979).

34 Volicer, B.J.; Burns, M.W.: Pre-existing correlates of hospital stress. Nursing Research 26: 408–415 (1977).

35 Wilson, J.F.: Behavioral preparation for surgery: benefit or harm? J. Behav. Med. 4: 79–102 (1981).

36 Johnston, M.: Dimensions of recovery from surgery. Int. Rev. Appl. Psychol. 33: 505–520 (1984).

37 Janis, I.L.: Psychological Stress (Wiley, New York, 1958).

38 Auerbach, S.M.: Trait-state anxiety and adjustment to surgery. J. Consult. Clin. Psychol. 34: 264–271 (1973).

39 Leventhal, H.: Findings and theory in the study of fear communications; in Berkowitz, Advances in Experimental Social Psychology, vol. 5 (Academic, New York, 1970).

40 Henry, J.P.; Stephens, P.M.: Stress, Health and the Social Environment: A Sociobiologic Approach. (Springer-Verlag, New York, 1977).

41 Johnson, J.E.: The effects of accurate expectations on the sensory and distress components of pain. J. Pers. Soc. Psychol. 27: 261–275 (1973).

42 Johnson, J.E.; Kirchhoff, K.T.; Endress, P.M.: Altering children's distress behavior during orthopaedic cast removal. Nursing Research 34: 404–410 (1975).

43 Johnson, J.E.; Rice, V.H.; Fuller, S.S.; Endress, M.P.: Sensory information, instruction in a coping strategy, and recovery from surgery. Res. Nursing Health 1: 4–17 (1978).

44 Johnson, J.E.; Fuller, S.S.; Endress, M.P.; Rice, V.H.: Altering patients' responses to surgery: an extension and replication. Res. Nursing Health 1: 111–121 (1978).

45 Fuller, S.S.; Endress, P.M.; Johnson, J.E.: The effects of cognitive and behavioral control on coping with an aversive health examination. J. Hum. Stress 4: 18–25 (1978).

46 Staite, S.A.: The effect of giving information about post-operative sensations on mood and pain in patients undergoing gynaecological surgery. (Unpublished M. Phil. Thesis, University of London, 1978).

47 Johnston, M.: Emotional distress immediately following surgery; in Tiller and Martin, Behavioral Medicine (Geigy, Melbourne, 1981).

48   Levesque, L.; Charlebois, M.: Anxiety, locus of control, and the effect of pre-operative teaching on patients' physical and emotional state. Nursing Papers 8: 11–26 (1977).

49   Mathews, A.; Ridgeway, V.: Personality and surgical recovery: a review. Br. J. Clin. Psychol. 2: 243–260 (1981).

50   Langer, E.; Janis, I.J.; Wolfer, J.A.: Reduction of psychological stress in surgical patients. J. exp. Soc. Psychol. 11: 155–165 (1975).

51   Meichenbaum, D.; Turk, D.; Burstein, S.: The nature of coping with stress; in Sarason and Spielberger, Stress Anxiety, vol. 2, pp. 337–360 (Wiley, New York, 1975).

52   Cohen, F.; Lazarus, R.S.: Coping with the stresses of illness; in Stone, Cohen and Adler, Health Psychology: A Handbook, pp. 217–254 (Jossey-Bass, San Francisco, 1979).

53   Ridgeway, V.; Matthews, A.M.: Psychological preparation for surgery: a comparison of methods. Br. J. Clin. Psychol. 21: 271–280 (1982).

54   Ray, C.: The surgical patient: psychological stress and coping resources; in Eiser, Social Psychology and Behavioral Medicine, pp. 483–507 (Wiley, London, 1981).

55   Miller, S.M.: When is a little information a dangerous thing? Coping with stressful events by monitoring versus blunting; in Levine and Ursin, Coping and Health, pp. 145–169 (Plenum Press, New York, 1980).

56   Auerbach, S.M.; Kilman, P.R.: Crisis intervention: a review of outcome research. Psychol. Bull. 84: 1189–1217 (1977).

57   Andrew, J.M.: Recovery from surgery with and without preparatory instruction for three coping styles. J. Pers. Soc. Psychol. 15: 223–226 (1970).

58   Ray, C.J.; Fitzgibbon, G.: Socially mediated reduction of stress in surgical patients; in Oborne, Gruneberg, Eiser, Research in Psychology and Medicine, pp. 321–327 (Academic, London, 1980).

59   Williams, J.G.L.; Jones, J.R.; Workhoven, M.N.; Williams, B.: The psychological control of pre-operative anxiety. Psychophysiol. 12: 50–54 (1975).

60   Bradley, C.: The contribution of psychological factors; in Watkins and Salo, Trauma, Stress and Immunity in Anaesthesia and Surgery (Butterworth, London, 1982).

61   Boore, J.R.P.: Prescription for Recovery. (Royal College of Nursing, London, 1978).

62   Kinney, M.R.: Effects of pre-operative teaching upon patients with differing modes of response to treatment stimuli. Int. J. Nurs. Stud. 14: 49–59 (1977).

63   Friedman, S.B.; Mason, J.W.; Hamburg, D.A.: Urinary 17 – hydroxycorticosteroid levels in parents of children with neoplastic disease. Psychosom. Med. 35: 364–376 (1964).

Marie Johnston, PhD, Senior Lecturer in Clinical Psychology, Royal Free Hospital School of Medicine, University of London, Pond Street, London NW3 2QG (England)

Adv. psychosom. Med., vol. 15, pp. 23–50 (Karger, Basel 1986)

Psychological Intervention with Surgical Patients: Evaluation Outcome

Malcolm Rogers, Peter Reich

Harvard Medical School, Brigham and Women's Hospital, Boston, Mass., USA

This chapter examines outcome measures following psychological intervention with surgical patients. Rather than examining the theoretical bases for post-surgical emotional outcomes, as is done on p. 1, this chapter is more clinically focused as it examines outcome data for a number of psychological interventions on surgical patients. For example, programmatic interventions are measured that impact: post-operative pain or narcotic use, duration of hospitalization, post-operative delirium, inter-operative states, post-operative vomiting, long-term adjustment, etc. The following case will help us to frame some of the psychological approaches and interventions used.

At the age of 58, Mrs. A. was filled with dread at the prospect of having both of her hips replaced. She had been struggling with chronic arthritis since the age of seven. Having been widowed for several years, and now on the eve of her youngest son's departure for college, she knew that being able to care for herself in the years ahead was of crucial importance. She managed to walk, albeit with a very awkward gait, yet her hips were so flexed that sitting was difficult and walking downstairs without assistance nearly impossible. Remaining self-sufficient had been an obsession since childhood. She remembered the terrible pangs of loneliness and isolation she felt as a teenager when confined to the hospital for almost one year. To this day, little things such as the sound of a light switch which the nurse flipped on each morning at six o'clock in her hospital room, brought back the dread of this period of confinement and helplessness.

Understandably she had trouble tolerating the thought of a similar confinement for hip surgery now. Giving up her mobility for even two weeks in the post-operative phase terrified her. Her rheumatologist became aware of the extent of this dread as the patient often refused a physical exam during her office visits. Somewhat reluctantly Mrs. A. agreed to accept a referral for psychiatric evaluation and treatment.

During the course of the next year, she met regularly with the psychiatrist to whom she had been referred. Fortunately, he was quite familiar with the orthopedic procedure and post-operative course to which she would be subjected. Many hours were spent in discussing memories of childhood experiences with her illness and prior hospitalizations. Despite her deformities, her determination and ego strengths were such that she was able to marry, to work for a period of time as an accountant, and finally to bear and raise two healthy children. She talked about the future and what it would be like without her two sons living at home. After six months of out-patient psychotherapy, it was clear that she viewed surgery as a foregone conclusion. The only issue that remained was how and when she could go through with it. She began to ask more questions about the surgery, the risks, the pain, the potential gains in her mobility, and always the questions would come back to the immediate post-operative period. The image of being confined to bed in pain and helplessly dependent upon the nurses kept recurring. Finally she was able to schedule a deadline for the surgery, carefully picking the most opportune time for her own as well as her sons' schedule.

Partly for her benefit and partly for the staff's education, she participated in a meeting along with several other patients and representatives from each department in the hospital who would be involved in each phase of her care. Present was another patient like herself who faced the prospect of surgery, and several patients who were at various post-operative stages, some up to one year after the completion of hip replacement surgery. At the meeting, an orthopedic surgeon, a physical therapist, an occupational therapist, a nurse, an anesthesiologist, a social worker, and a psychiatrist each spoke briefly about the expected course of a hospitalization for a total hip replacement.

Eventually the day of the surgery arrived. Both hips were replaced with a 10 day interval between the two operations. Throughout her hospitalization she was followed closely by the same psychiatrist who had been treating her as an out-patient. On the eve of both procedures, she was frightened especially about the post-operative pain, but her anxiety was manageable both by her own efforts and by the staff working with her. The experience of the first operation made the second one easier. As a result of the surgery, she was able to continue to live independently and travel with considerably less difficulty.

Most psychiatrists involved in consultation liaison activities have encountered patients like Mrs. A. They believe that psychological intervention helped the patient through, perhaps in reducing the level of anxiety both pre- and post-operatively, perhaps in reducing pain and discomfort post-operatively, and even perhaps in reducing post-operative complications. Indeed, as in this case, the surgery might never have occurred had it not been for the psychiatric intervention.

Many patients now insist on some type of pre-operative preparation. The public is better informed generally about health care and medical practice. They are more inclined to ask questions, and less inclined to defer to the unquestioned authority of the doctor and other health care providers. In some pre-surgical situations such a child birth, formalized preparatory sessions have become an accepted standard of practice. Legal and ethical pressures surrounding informed consent have required that physicians spell out in detail the consequences and risks associated with any surgical procedure, although completion of the written form in no way substitutes for a real discussion. Current nursing practice, at least in major medical centers, has included pre-operative and post-operative teaching as a routine part of hospital care for surgical patients.

Intuitive sense indicates that pre-operative psychological intervention and preparation is good surgical care. The aim of this chapter is to examine the evidence supporting this approach. Is pre-operative preparation cost effective – a question posed nowadays with increasing frequency? Does it decrease post-operative complications, such as delirium or infection? Does it shorten the post-operative course and decrease the overall length of stay? Does it facilitate long-term rehabilitation? Although it is a harder question to answer, does it reduce the immediate psychological suffering and perhaps long range psychological consequences of the procedure? There have, in fact, been an impressive number of research studies which have examined these questions and in many cases provided affirmative answers.

The Impact of Surgery

Before examining the results of these studies in detail, it is worth considering briefly some of the known emotional and physiological concomitants of surgery. The impact, of course, varies widely according to the procedure, its meaning to the patient, the personality of the patient, and the state of the underlying disease. The surgery may occur on an emergency basis in a general atmosphere of crisis and confusion for the patient and family and sometimes for the surgeon. Or, at the other end of the spectrum, it may occur as a carefully planned elective and voluntary procedure. No matter which, there is general agreement that surgery constitutes a major psychological stress.

Physiological Stress

The stress of anticipating surgery has been discussed on p. 1. One outcome of pre-surgical stress is the elevation of adrenal corticosteroid levels. Adults hospitalized for thoracic surgery have elevated plasma steroid concentrations prior to the surgery, with those patients having higher steroid concentrations tending to display behavior suggestive of states of marked discomfort post-operatively [1]. The evening prior to surgery, a pulse of cortisol secretion occurs six to tenfold greater than found in pre-operative controls, triggered consistently by preoperative preparation (shaving complete chest, abdomen, leg; antiseptic wash; and enema [2]). The stark reality of the pre-operative preparation presumably disrupts the psychological defense of denial. Elevations in growth hormone as well as adrenal gluco-corticoid activity have also been shown in patients preparing to undergo cardiac catheterization [3] and in children undergoing open heart surgery, not only on the day before surgery but also on the day of return from the intensive care unit [4]. Studies of serum cortisol in women awaiting breast tumor biopsy indicate that the effectiveness of psychological defense mechanisms is the critical predictor of the adrenal glucocorticoid response to the stress of hospitalization and anticipated surgery [5]. In children undergoing elective surgery, cortisol levels both before hospitalization and in the hospital were highest in those children whose coping capacity was lowest; yet 2 weeks prior to admission to the hospital there was no correlation between coping and cortisol levels. Those children who use defenses of intellectualization, or flexible mixed defenses, showed lower levels of cortisol than those children using more primative defenses such as denial, projection or rigid defensive postures [7]. Thus, a number of studies have concluded that it is not simply the stress of surgery per se, but how the operation is perceived and coped with that determines the level of endocrine response.

The degree of elevation in adrenal gluco-corticoids may have some specific consequences in the post-operative course. While a certain degree of elevation in this response may represent a physiologically adaptive response, higher levels may increase the risk of immunosuppression and post-operative infection. Immunosuppression is known to occur post-operatively [8].

Psychological Stress

Surgery is commonly regarded as a psychologically threatening experience for which an adaptive response is required. As mentioned on p. 1,
Janis was among the first to articulate the view that a moderate level of pre-
operative anxiety was adaptive [9]. Patients at either ends of the spectrum –
either those showing an absence of anxiety or those showing overwhelming
levels of anxiety – were thought to be at risk. Subsequent investigators have
questioned this basic model, since patients with low fear ratings have more
favorable outcomes than either the high or moderate fear patients, based on
a number of recovery variables [10]. The issue turns on the effectiveness of
individual coping strategies and the variability of coping styles according to
personality differences (about which we will have more to say later). There
have been numerous reports of psychological morbidity following surgery
due to unrealistic expectations on the part of patients [13], post-traumatic
stress reactions [14], and a range of other unanticipated psychological complications [15].

The outcome of psychological stress experienced during hospitalization
for surgery can be seen for some patients in the immediate post-operative
period. For other patients, the outcome of surgical stress may be observed
only after hospital discharge, with the onset of behavioral and emotional
problems. These have been best documented in children. In one early study,
approximately 10–35% of children undergoing tonsillectomy and adenoidectomy developed subsequent behavior problems [11]. In a similar study, 57
percent of a group of children who had had forced induction of anesthesia,
compared to 40 percent who had quiet induction, developed behavioral
symptoms months later – such as temper tantrums, fearfulness and bedwet-
ting [12].

Outcome of Psychologic Intervention in Surgical Patients

Unfortunately there is no simple or single measure of 'successful recovery from surgery', as was initially discussed on p. 1. Many different measures
have been used, such as: length of hospital stay, use of medications for pain,
patients' own subjective reports of pain, other 'satisfaction' measures, and
various other physiological parameters. Typically correlations among these
variables have been low [16]. Most studies have measured several different
outcome variables. We have organized this review of different psychological

intervention studies around specific outcome variables, concentrating on those in which the demonstration of efficacy is clearest.

Pain Reduction

Twenty years ago a team of anesthesiologists headed by *Lawrence Egbert* investigated the effects of pre-operative psychological intervention on post-operative pain and medication use [18]. In one experiment *Egbert* et al. demonstrated that a five minute visit by an anesthesiologist the night before the operation, outlining the plan of care on the day of surgery reduced significantly pre-operative anxiety. In fact, calmness in patients just before the induction of anesthesia was associated more with this 5 minute interview than the administration of pentobarbital. In a second study approximately 100 patients undergoing elective abdominal surgery received such a pre-operative visit from an anesthesiologist the night before surgery [19]. One half of this group was randomly assigned to the experimental group, to which additional information was provided about post-operative pain. These patients were informed about post-operative pain in terms of its severity and duration and reassured about it normality. The anesthesiologist went on to explain that the methods of pain relief available post-operatively included both analgesics and relaxation. Patients were told that the pain was caused by straining of the wound, and that if they were careful to not move the area of the wound, they would have little or no pain. They were also told how to breathe and cough and turn from side to side in a way that would reduce their abdominal pain. Fifty-seven of these patients were rated post-operatively by an independent observer who noted that the specially prepared patients seemed more comfortable post-operatively and also used one-half as much morphine for the five days following surgery. It should be stated however, that during the recovery period the specially prepared experimental group continued to receive special visits and information, including specific instruction in coughing. Thus, the groups were treated differently post-operatively as well, perhaps producing subtle pressure to use less narcotic medication. Other studies have also shown that coughing instructions per se have been associated with reduced analgesic medication and earlier discharge [20]. In any case, the authors interpreted their study as showing the importance of the placebo response, and the potent psychotherapeutic power possessed by physicians.

In the years since the *Egbert* study, the results of studies of the effects of psychological intervention on post-operative pain and analgesic use have been varied. Some investigations have failed to show any reduction in post-operative pain or analgesic medication usage. For example, a study by *Johnson* et al. [21] attempted to prepare female patients undergoing elective abdominal surgery by exploring their thoughts and feelings about the impending operation as well as giving patients advice about breathing, turning and surgery. Pain reports did not differ between the two groups. *Lindemann and Stetzer* studied the effect of pre-operative visits by operating theater nurses who provided patients undergoing non-emergency surgical procedures with greater information about the surgery. Outcome was measured in terms of nursing care in the OR, patient anxiety and post-operative welfare. A significant reduction in post-operative anxiety was found in patients undergoing minor, but not major, surgical trauma [22]. There was no correlation between psychological intervention and the amount of analgesics used within 48 hours post-operatively. In an earlier study the same investigators had failed to find a positive correlation between structured pre-operative teaching of breathing exercises by nurses and post-operative analgesic use, although post-operative respiratory function was significantly improved and the length of hospital stay was reduced significantly as well [23].

Another negative finding was reported by *Surman*, who attempted to improve the post-operative course in adults undergoing cardiac surgery with one or more therapeutic interviews pre-operatively. The interviews were intended to be supportive and to clear up any misconceptions about the forthcoming surgery. These interviewers also included teaching of a simple auto-hypnotic technique. This intervention had no effect on post-operative pain or quantity of analgesic usage [24]. Similarly in another study of pre-operative teaching by nurses in adults undergoing major surgery, no reduction in post-operative use of analgesics was noted [25].

However there has also been some impressive evidence in support of *Egbert's* earlier observations. One study showed that small group therapy sessions the evening before surgery and additional 15–60 minute sessions with the nurse on the morning of surgery reduced the amount of post-operative analgesics used during the second and third post-operative days [26]. Improvement occurred in several other outcomes measures: decreased anxiety the morning of surgery, less urinary retention, less anesthesia, more rapid return to oral intake and earlier discharge. *Langer* et al. showed that a 20 minute pre-operative session with a psychologist reduced the percentage of subjects requesting sedatives and the total number of analgesics used. A special coping technique was taught which entailed the cognitive reappraisal of anxiety-provoking events, calm 'self-talk', and cognitive control through selective attention. This technique was more efficacious than providing information alone [27]. A more time-consuming method was employed by *Fortin and Kirouac*, involving pre-operative education and training by nurses in one session per week starting 15–20 days before hospitalization [28]. This intervention led to a significant reduction in the amount of pain present at the time of discharge.

A much briefer, focused approach was used in a study by *Flaherty* et al. [29]. They used a relaxation technique taught by a nurse pre-operatively. Pain and distress were measured during the patient's first attempt to get out of bed after surgery. This intervention significantly reduced the amount of post-operative Demerol required as well as the reported intensity and distress from the incisional pain. Furthermore, it also significantly lowered post-operative respiratory rate.

Although the results are not always consistent, it would appear that interventions ranging from reassurance alone, to the teaching of special coping strategies and relaxation techniques, and group therapy, have all been shown to reduce post-operative pain experience and analgesic usage. Some differences in outcome result from the differences in the type and duration of intervention, and from differences in outcome measures and patient populations. (And in some of the studies, such as *Egbert's*, continued post-operative intervention occurred.) In general, nurses have been more aggressive than physicians in implementing these pre-operative interventions.

Shortened Duration of Hospitalization

Almost all studies of psychological intervention pre-operatively have studied more than one outcome measure post-operatively. Many have studied the length of hospitalization, a measure of particular importance currently because of efforts to contain the costs of hospitalization. A cost/benefit ratio analysis has become an important way of evaluating many medical interventions. Few would question the importance of pre-operative psychological preparation if it were shown consistently to reduce the length of hospitalization and thereby reduce substantially the cost of medical treatment. And, in fact, there is substantial evidence from the studies which have been undertaken to indicate that such intervention does indeed reduce the length of hospitalization. In a recent review of these studies, *Mumford* et al. have summarized much of the available data [30]. In examining 14 controlled studies (13 of them relating to pre-operative intervention and 1 of them to intervention in myocardial infarction), these authors concluded that an average reduction of 2.37 days of hospitalization occurred in the intervention group. Looking at the studies in total, the data were based on approximately 2000 intervention and control patients. Eight of the thirteen studies showed a difference of one or more days, the largest difference being five days. Five studies failed to show any difference. None of these studies were blind, however, in the sense that the staff caring for the patient post-operatively was unaware of pre-operative intervention. Therefore there may have been a subtle bias in the direction of speeding up the process of post-operative rehabilitation for earlier discharge. The effect of being measured thus may well have been a subtle post-operative intervention in addition to the pre-operative intervention.

The bias toward earlier, more appropriate discharge was certainly present in one other recent study showing the clinical and cost benefits of liaison psychiatry in elderly patients with recent emergency surgery for hip fractures [31]. In this study a liaison psychiatrist participated in the post-operative care of a group of elderly patients. Their clinical outcomes were compared with a control group of patients not treated by a liaison psychiatrist. A total of 24 patients were seen within 72 hours of admission and followed and treated by the psychiatrist until discharged. The liaison psychiatrist worked closely with the house staff, nursing staff, social service department, physiotherapy staff, attending staff, family and friends. The treated patients were discharged on the average 12 days before the control group. Twice as many patients in the treatment group returned home rather than being discharged to a nursing home or some other health related institution. The authors point out that these two variables may be related in that the patients being transferred to nursing homes may have had longer hospitalizations, partly because they were waiting for nursing home beds to become available. The raised expectations and energy on the part of the entire staff would appear to be able to improve outcome, and may have been a factor operating in the studies cited above.

Reduction of Post-Operative Delirium

Post-operative delirium has been identified as a significant post-operative complication in patients undergoing open heart surgery [32–34], cataract surgery [35], in elderly patients undergoing all types of surgery [36, 37] and in patients undergoing total joint replacement [38]. (Delirium is discussed more fully on p. 51 and on p. 124). Estimates of the incidence have varied but in many series approximately 25% of the patients undergoing operative procedures have developed post-operative delirium. Many risk factors and etiologic mechanisms have been identified including: advanced age, pre-operative cognitive deficit, pre-operative anxiety and personality factors, the magnitude of the physiologic disruption in surgery, time under anesthesia, the role of sedative-hypnotic medication and alcohol withdrawal, sleep deprivation, and sensory deprivation. In most situations a single clear etiologic factor is difficult to identify. One often postulates a multi-factorial etiology in a susceptible host with reduced threshhold for the occurrence of post-operative delirium.

Interestingly some of the investigative efforts to clarify the mechanisms for post-operative delirium have inadvertently provided pre-operative, and in some cases post-operative, interventions which have themselves altered the responses being investigated. For example, *Lazarus* et al. found that one interview conducted 2–3 days prior to surgery reduced the incidence of immediate post-operative psychosis by 50% or more [39], although other factors, such as a special teaching session for the recovery room staff, may also have played a role. In another study, *Kornfeld* et al. discovered unexpectedly that a single interview with a psychiatrist pre-operatively reduced by 50% the incidence of post-cardiotomy delirium [32]. In the *Kornfeld* study, patients who demonstrated personality traits of dominance, aggressiveness and self-assuredness were at greater risk of experiencing post-operative delirium. These studies have also indicated that the incidence of post-operative delirium as evaluated by retrospective chart analysis is approximately 50% of the real incidence based on post-operative clinical evaluation.

A single one hour therapeutic interview before surgery was also found by *Layne and Udofsky* to result in a 50% reduction in post-operative psychosis following open heart surgery. The intervention produced no difference in post-operative mortality however [40]. Using a modified systematic desensitization technique in patients undergoing open heart surgery, *Aiken and Henricks* were able to reduce significantly the incidence of post-operative psychosis [41], although their control patients operated on a year or two earlier were exposed to less physiologic stress during the operation itself.

On the other hand, *Surman* failed to show any significant decrease in post-operative delirium in patients undergoing cardiac surgery by using a similar intervention of one or more therapeutic interviews including the teaching of auto-hypnosis for a 60–90 minute period [24]. However, in this study the experimental group differed from the control group in that subjects in the experimental group were more likely to have had prior psychiatric treatment and on the average had been medically ill for four years longer than the control group. Interestingly in spite of the negative results in terms of post-operative delirium, their intervention did significantly reduce: the amount of time spent in the intensive care unit, by 17 hours; intubation time, by 19 hours; and overall time in hospital, by 3.6 days.

A recent study may provide a possible explanation [42]. Adults admitted for cardiac surgery in the experimental group were simply advised of the possible unusual perceptual disturbances associated with delirium which might occur in the post-operative period. Although the intervention group showed no statistical decrease in the amount of delirium compared to the non-intervention group, nonetheless those patients reported feeling significantly more comfortable and in control when confronted with these unusual experiences, compared to the non-intervention group.

Physiological Measures

Other physiological parameters have been included as outcome measurements of pre-operative or pre-anesthesia interventions. These measurements have been made: immediately prior to the induction of anesthesia, intra-operatively, immediately post-operatively in the recovery room, and throughout the post-operative course.

Intra-Operative Effects

Although this has been discussed already in other sections relating to pain and emotional states, the intraoperative state of the patient becomes even more critically important when the patient remains awake during the procedure and, in fact, is required to cooperate. For example, in endoscopy, cardiac catheterization or dental treatment, the patient is moderately sedated but nevertheless needs to be a participant in the procedure itself. Psychological preparation prior to gastrointestinal endoscopy has resulted in significantly fewer tranquilizers being required for the endoscopic procedure [43]. Moreover, a description of the sensations which were typically experienced in the procedure, as opposed to technical information about it, resulted in less restlessness and lower heart rate during the examination as well as a lower rate of tension during the passage of the endoscope tube [43]. Numerous studies have demonstrated the beneficial effect of preparation in dental treatment [45, 46]. Similar efforts have been made in preparation for childbirth [47]. It is now common practice for expectant mothers and their spouses to undergo a series of preparatory sessions involving breathing exercises and information about the typical course of events during delivery. Cooperation during cardiac catheterization has been shown to be improved by preparing the patient with both specific information and emotional support during two sessions – one the day before the procedure and one on the day of surgery [48]. The largest effect in this study was in the reduction of psychotropic medication required during the procedure itself.

Recovery Room Effects

The degree of post-operative vomiting in the recovery room has been shown to be reduced from 54% to 16% by encouragement and close one-to-one monitoring from surgical nurses [49]. In this study, a nurse visited adult women about to undergo gynecologic surgery and remained with the patient while she was in the recovery room.

Other Post-Operative Effects

Alterations in respiratory function have been noted to occur following pre-operative psychologic intervention. For example, patients undergoing major abdominal surgery received training in a relaxation technique [29]. During their first attempt to get out of bed six to eight hours after surgery, the experimental group had a significantly lower respiratory rate than the control group. More specific and sophisticated measures of respiratory function, however, have failed to find any significant correlation between intervention and pulmonary function. *Archuleta*, in a study of adults undergoing major surgery, arranged for pre-operative teaching by a nurse plus five minutes of post-operative reinforcement in the experimental group. However, this study failed to demonstrate any changes in: forced vital capacity, maximal mid-expiratory flow or forced expiration volume at one second [25]. Similarly, *Felton* et al. using pre-operative information provided by a nurse together with photographs and films with adults undergoing major surgery for the first time, failed to show any improvement in ventilatory function at either 24, 48 or 72 hours post-operatively [50]. However, a study by *Lindemann and Van Aernan* represents one striking exception to these results [23]. In their study, structured pre-operative teaching by nurses for adults undergoing chest and abdominal surgery resulted in significantly improved maximal expiratory flow rates and vital capacities measured post-operatively. In this situation, pre-operative teaching involved specific instructions about coughing techniques to be used post-operatively. This study provides good evidence for the necessity of carefully defining the outcome measurement in relation to the pre-operative intervention. In this case, the specificity of the pre-operative intervention did produce a significant effect on the post-operative measure of these same specific physiological parameters. We will say more about the range of intervention techniques used below.

In terms of cardiovascular effects, the more non-specific intervention employed by *Felton* et al. [50], namely, pre-operative intervention by a nurse using informational photographs and films, did reduce significantly the incidence of heart or circulatory complications in their experimental group. Interestingly, the therapeutic communication approach by a nurse lasting approximately the same length of time appeared to have the most dramatic effect in reducing heart or circulatory complications post-operatively. *Schmitt and Wooldridge* also found that small group therapy sessions the evening before surgery did reduce post-operative blood pressures [26]. Interestingly, these authors also found that the same interventions increased significantly the ability of experimental subjects to void post-operatively and, to a lesser extent, improved their ability to resume oral intake. Others have not found a significant change in post-operative pulse rate or blood pressure [29], and *Surman's* study of adults undergoing cardiac surgery failed to show that pre-operative psychologic intervention, which included both therapeutic interviews and auto-hypnosis, had any effect on incidence of cardiac failure or arrhythmia post-operatively [24]. However, as mentioned before, his experimental patients were more likely to have had a prior psychiatric history and had been medically ill for longer than the controls.

A variety of other outcome measures have been used. For example, several assessments of physical rehabilitation have been made. In one study, nine patients were prepared with hypnosis prior to knee surgery coupled with the suggestions that they would: sleep well after surgery, be less bothered by post-operative pain, and would be able to exercise their knees immediately after surgery [51]. The prepared patients had a significantly shortened period required for rehabilitation post-operatively and in fact were discharged significantly earlier. Other studies have shown that inpatient ambulatory activity and activities of daily living, including the capacity to return to work earlier, were significantly improved in a group of adults undergoing major surgery that received pre-operative education by nurses starting two to three weeks before hospitalization [52]. In a similar manner, encouragement from surgical residents pre- and post-operatively was found to reduce the need for post-operative urinary bladder catheterization from 18% to 2% [53].

Some other interesting outcome variables have been investigated in looking at the effects of presurgical psychologic preparation. *Florell's* study included measurements not only of length of hospitalization and narcotic use but also of number of calls for assistance and number of lines written in nursing notes as well as 'physiological responses' [54]. In this study, the experimental patients, compared to the control population, were shown to have fewer calls for assistance from the nurses, less written about them in fewer lines of nurses' notes, and lowered physiologic responses than the control population.

Psychologic Measures

Intuition would suggest that post-operative recovery, length of hospitalization, pain, and physiological parameters would all be positively correlated with good emotional health. On the other hand, correlations between independent outcome variables is known to be poor, and even though dysphoric emotional states may occur during the post-operative period, they may not directly interfere with the immediate post-operative recovery. Nevertheless dysphoric emotional states may have some long-term consequences for rehabilitation, quality of life and follow-up medical care.

Short-Term Effects

Intuition notwithstanding, the actual data available concerning the short-term psychological effects of pre-operative intervention present a somewhat more confusing picture. First of all, in some major studies in which no specific psychologic intervention was employed, the degree of pre-operative fear and anxiety was not correlated with any aspect of post-operative recovery [15, 55]. Much of this debate had stemmed from *Janis'* initial claim for the importance of the 'work of worrying' in the patient's own internal process of psychologic preparation for surgery. *Ray and Fitzgibbon,* on the other hand, suggested that one can make a distinction between positive affects, such as arousal and vigilance, and simple emotionality or stress per se, which they feel may have a negative impact [55].

In any event, several studies have looked in detail at post-operative emotional states following psychologic intervention (as reviewed on p. 1). A variety of psychologic measures have been used including: mood self-assessment scales, measurements of distress during hospitalization by nurses, measurements of cooperation recorded by nursing staff, measurements of personality, such as inner-directedness (closely related to the current concept of locus of control), and physicians' rating of patient depression and anxiety [9, 17, 48, 50, 56–58]. Most of these studies have shown some significant positive correlations between intervention and positive affective states immediately pre-operatively, but these correlations are rather weak during the days after surgery. For example, cardiac patients undergoing catheterization who were specifically informed of the procedure and given emotional support beforehand showed very mild but consistently improved outcomes in measures of well-being, happiness, fear, helplessness and anger [48]. *Felton* et al. found similar modest changes on a mood scale. However they found a much more powerful effect in terms of the patients' sense of inner-directedness and self-regard following their intervention, which consisted of pre-operative information given by a nurse supplemented with photographs and films [50]. A self-report measure of anxiety on the morning of surgery was also significantly reduced in a prepared group of males undergoing elective surgery [26].

The capacity of psychologic intervention to reduce fear and anxiety immediately before an operation is perhaps most clearly evidenced in several studies on children [60]. (Reactions to surgery in children is covered on p. 69). Some of the most creative types of intervention have been utilized in the preparation of children for surgery, such as puppet therapy and role playing. The effects of these creative interventions are often clearly demonstrable in children, not only on a short-term but also on a long-term basis. For example, if children are prepared pre-operatively then: willingness to return to a hospital 30 days post-operatively, adequacy of sleep, fear of doctors, fear of leaving mother and crying have in several studies of long-term follow-up been shown to improve significantly [59, 60].

Long-Term Effects

While a number of long-term measures of psychologic and behavioral functioning are shown to be improved in children who received intervention prior to surgery, there are few studies of long-term outcome measures in adults. This would appear to be a major gap in the literature. Many of the surgical procedures in adults, for example, joint-replacement surgery, require months and perhaps close to a year before the full physical benefits can be experienced. Post-operative depressions often develop after discharge from the hospital, particularly when unexpected incapacitation occurs or the patient's prior expectations are not in agreement with post-operative reality. (P. 200 reviews the psychological sequalae of limb amputation.) Indeed, most patients who have been chronically disabled and undergo surgery which can affect their level of disability do experience a period of emotional crisis in adaptation to this changed level of functioning and self-definition.

This issue of long-term outcome becomes particularly important not only for joint replacement surgery but also for adults undergoing coronary artery bypass grafts. Some earlier evidence has indicated that despite improvements in somatic symptomatology and physiologic measures, a patient's capacity to resume work is less than would be anticipated [61]. One might wonder whether long-term post-operative adjustment in terms of work, interpersonal relationships especially with spouse, sexual relationships and leisure time activities might be improved by careful pre- and post-operative preparation. Indeed, this kind of preparation need not be limited to the pre-operative period but might more appropriately focus on the post-operative period in preparation for discharge. Much effort has already gone into the rehabilitation of patients suffering an acute myocardial infarction with noticeable benefits [62].

Intervention Techniques

We will consider briefly the kinds of psychologic intervention techniques utilized, and how they differ from one another.

Informational

Information is, of course, an enormously powerful tool. In general, most patients anticipating a hospital experience and surgery are as frightened by the unknown and potential loss of control as by any of the physical dimensions such as pain. Information may be provided by many different people ranging from the surgeon, to the nurse involved in post-operative care, to the recovery room nurse, to the anesthesiologist, or to the physical therapist who may be involved with the patient post-operatively. Thus, many different types of professionals are involved in different phases of the patient's pre- and post-surgical care. Information may be delivered in person, or it may be packaged on film or videotape. It may be presented individually or to a group. The manner in which the information is provided and at what level of detail is relevant to the category of psychotherapeutic relationship considered below. Clinical experience and conventional wisdom would suggest that patients should be provided with as much information as they express a need for and conversely should not be overwhelmed with uninvited details.

Some experimental evidence bears out this clinical wisdom. For example, there is evidence that experimental electric shocks, for which adequate preparation is given, are experienced as less aversive and noxious [63]. Other work has suggested the importance of information in reducing uncertainty, and hence anxiety and distress from internal sensations, be they pain or other, which are likely to be encountered post-operatively. *Johnson,* for example, has been a particularly strong advocate of preparing patients by explaining in detail the internal sensations which are likely to be experienced post-operatively [21]. In her comparison of two different information techniques – one involving information about what the patient would experience, the other involving technical information about the procedure (e.g. endoscopy) – the former was found to have a more calming effect. *Mumford's* review [30] suggests that most interventions, even when not matched for the subject's particular needs, are effective in reducing length of hospitalization and favorably impacting several other outcome measures. Most of these interventions involve the provision of information; in many of the studies, the presentation of information was the sole intervention made. In some cases, the information was quite specific. For example, *Lindemann's* interventions in teaching pre-operative patients how to cough effectively were shown to be associated with improved ventilatory function post-operatively [23].

Hypnosis

Hypnotherapy has been used as the primary intervention technique in a number of studies. It has been used either by the operating surgeon or by a research assistant on a one time basis; it has also been taught as a self-hypnotic technique prior to surgery, thus presumably used post-operatively by the patient. For the most part, hypnosis has been used as a method of relieving pain, thus reducing the amount of anesthesia needed during surgery or the amount of post-operative analgesic medication used. *Bonilla* et al. utilized this technique in adult males undergoing knee surgery. Their intervention groups required less post-operative analgesia and had a shorter average rehabilitation time (27 vs 46 days) [51]. In most patients, hypnosis was

performed one day before surgery with the following post-hypnotic suggestions: 1. that the patient would not fear the operation and would have a good
night's sleep on the evening prior to surgery; 2. that he/she would be aware
of the inevitable post-operative pain but would not be bothered by it; and
3. that he/she would be able to exercise the knee immediately after surgery.
Kolouch also utilized this technique to shorten effectively the length of hospitalization and reduce analgesic use [64]. In another study, one or two sessions of hypnosis pre-operatively reduced the amount of narcotic utilization
and was associated with improved mood post-operatively [65]. One very
interesting account comes from *Gruen* who prepared himself for cardiac surgery by using self-relaxation and self-suggestion and was able to reduce his
requirement for narcotics and recover at a better than average rate [66]. On
the other hand, *Surman,* using the technique of auto-hypnosis together with
one or more therapeutic interviews, was unable to show an effect on post-operative complications or pain medication use, although the experimental
group was discharged an average of four days earlier. One can assume that
different patients will have different degrees of acceptance of this technique
and varying capacity to respond to it for pain control or other purposes.
Kolouch found that both the magnitude of surgery and the presence of
unspecified 'personality problems' in patients diminished the usefulness of
hypnosis [64].

Relaxation

The specific use of relaxation training as a presurgical intervention technique has been generally successful either alone or in combination with other
techniques. The first positive response reported was in a study by *Aiken and
Henricks* [41]. Adult males undergoing heart surgery were exposed to a
modified, systematic desensitization approach, presented by a cardiac nurse
specialist in combination with a 15-minute tape-recorded relaxation exercise.
This intervention did reduce significantly the amount of post-operative psychosis. However, patients receiving the relaxation had somewhat less serious
operations than did the control patients and required less time under anesthesia and on cardiopulmonary bypass. Finally, a recent study by *Flagherty
and Fitzpatrick* taught patients undergoing abdominal surgery to use the relaxation technique of their first attempt to get out of bed. Patients using this
technique required less post-operative Demerol and complained less of incisional pain. They also had less change in pulse and respiratory rate on their

first attempt to get out of bed [29]. However, two other studies using relaxation as a pre-operative preparation failed to show significant differences in length of hospitalization or pain control [68, 69] although in one study post-operative anxiety was reduced.

Both this technique and other techniques taught to patients for post-operative use undoubtedly increase their sense of control and power in the situation. *Wilson* has looked at the interaction between this technique (as well as other techniques) and personality style and found that less frightened patients benefited more from relaxation techniques than did very frightened patients [67].

Supportive Psychotherapeutic Relationship

In most cases, the psychotherapeutic relationship also includes other modalities, such as the dispensing of important information or the teaching of a specific technique. For example, in *Egbert's* classic study, in which patients were visited the night before surgery by the anesthesiologist, reassurance as well as information were important parts of the intervention [19]. This simple intervention, which was a landmark study, reduced significantly the amount of pain and post-operative morphine used as well as the number of days in the hospital. Perhaps the most dramatic report of the power of even a brief psychotherapeutic relationship was offered by *Dumas and Leonard* [49]. Post-operative vomiting was reduced by a nurse visiting a patient one hour before surgery and remaining with the patient until the moment of anesthesia. The continuity of a relationship with a health professional interested in the patient's emotional state is probably an under-appreciated factor in outcome results.

Brief pre-operative interviewing with a psychiatrist or psychologist has been shown to reduce the incidence of post-operative psychosis in several different studies [29, 32, 40]. It is unclear to what extent these therapeutic interviews included some information about the possible development of post-operative delirium, which would have enabled the patient to identify delirium post-operatively and to cope with it. Continuity in this situation provides familiarity with people and surroundings which may help to obviate the occurrence of disorientation and other signs of delirium.

Submitting to surgery requires placing unusual trust in the surgeon, anesthesiologist, and special care nurses. It tends to mobilize powerful transference reactions which can be utilized in the interest of improving the post-operative course.

Other Supportive/Education Approaches

Many specialities have come to rely on nurse clinical specialists to do a great deal of pre-operative teaching in the context of a continuing relationship, although the specifics of the contact are not well-documented in the literature. At the Brigham and Women's Hospital in Boston for example, there are nurse clinical specialists in orthopedic surgery, kidney transplantation surgery, cardiac surgery and for the care of ostomy patients, to name only a few. Despite the fact that this approach has become standard clinical procedure in a number of settings, the special skills and knowledge base which such a clinician should bring to pre-operative patient contacts have not been delineated or disseminated sufficiently. In good practice, a patient scheduled to undergo surgical correction for scoliosis might be shown the kind of brace to be worn post-operatively, and might be led on a tour of relevant clinical areas to be utilized during hospitalization. These interventions might occur over a number of visits, actually starting months before the scheduled surgery.

Another supportive/educational technique (often informal) is peer counseling. Other patients at various post-operative stages and even pre-operatively, may have some contact with the identified patient. The value of contact with patients who have undergone successful surgery cannot be overestimated. Patients are frequently too intimidated to ask their various health professionals many of their most pressing questions. With a fellow patient, they may more comfortably identify what their preexisting, particular anxieties may be.

Clearly, the concept of preparation for surgery must acknowledge the extraordinarily different circumstances associated with many operations. Some operations, for example, require only preparation for the fear of anesthesia and perhaps post-operative pain; otherwise post-operatively nothing else is specifically required of the patient. However, after certain procedures, such as joint replacement surgery, there are enormous demands placed on the patient to undergo physical therapy and perhaps to exercise in a more vigorous fashion than has been the case for months or years. Particular post-operative phobias or depression may be triggered in these situations [15]. Some procedures are associated with special deformities or assaults on body image such as ostomies or amputations; and others, such as surgery for suspected malignancies may be associated with post-operative fear of death. Many of these special situations are described elsewhere in this book (limb amputation, p. 200; mastectomy, p. 109; penile implants, p. 212; gastric bypass, p. 140; renal transplant, p. 167) and accordingly require individualized approaches. Beyond that, of course, the unique needs of different kinds of patients with quite different personality styles and coping abilities become a crucial consideration, and one which underscores the importance of the relationship. Information has been described as something to be given to the patient. It is equally important for most patients to be able to give information about themselves and their families. Being understood as people by their health care providers facilitates cooperation and hence convalescence from surgery.

Differences in Personality, Coping Style and Intervention Strategy

The possibility exists that the efficacy of psychologic interventions could be significantly enhanced by tailoring them to the particular personality style of the patient. The evidence presented thus far shows that the length of hospitalization can be reduced by using a relatively rigid intervention technique without reference to the personality style of the patient. Certainly broad differences in preexisting emotional states of patients about to undergo surgery have been noted. Several investigators have wondered whether patients who use denial as a coping style in order to avoid the 'work of worrying' as described by *Janis* might be harmed by pre-operative preparation. In fact, there have been some reports of negative effects particularly in patients designated as deniers or avoiders, who generally have a slower recovery anyway. *Andrew* reported that patients classified as 'deniers' responded to behavioral preparation with increased use of pain medication [70]. There have also been reports of increased frequency of complaints [71] and increased physiologic evidence of stress [72].

Such untoward results raise the question about why certain interventions work and for what kinds of personality styles. Is it that preparation allows patients to rehearse mentally how they will cope with the post-operative situation and thus to elicit preexisting coping skills? Or perhaps using a behavioral framework, as in the desensitization experience, it works by extinguishing conditioned fear responses. And even if it failed to extinguish a conditioned fear response completely for the current surgery, it might prevent the subsequent development of a phobia towards hospitals or medical care. Or perhaps the benefit is from the reduction of uncertainty and the psychological benefit of having a predictable environment. Perhaps the reduction in isolation, or the sense of being understood and cared for in a relationship, is the most important ingredient. We are a long way from having answered these questions specifically although, in many ways, the surgical situation provides an ideal opportunity for the exploration and evaluation of the efficacy of different psychotherapeutic techniques.

A few investigators have begun to seek answers to these questions by direct study. *Klos* et al. investigated 50 patients who were scheduled for cholecystectomy [73]. All patients were given information on the expected sequence of events on the day of surgery and instructions in post-operative self-care activities. Their findings indicated that there was a differential effect of this information depending on the patient's level of pre-operative fear. High fear patients benefited most from the intervention, which came either in the form of a pamphlet and/or a nurse visit. Patients in the high pre-operative fear group who received either the pamphlet or the pamphlet and a nurse visit had shorter post-operative hospitalizations, switched from injected to oral medication sooner, scored higher on an index of energy and movement, and rated their appetites as better when compared with patients in either the nurse visit alone group or the control group. However, among those who scored low in pre-operative fear, patients in the control group had better recoveries from surgery than patients who received pre-operative information. The results of this study are not entirely consistent with other reports. However, it does clearly demonstrate a differential effect of the intervention according to the affective state of the patient.

Another interesting experiment was reported by *Wilson* [67] on patients undergoing either elective cholecystectomy or hysterectomy, prepared either with training in muscle relaxation or with information about sensations which they would experience post-operatively. Relaxation reduced hospital stay, pain, and medication for pain and increased strength, energy, and post-operative epinephrine levels. Information was also shown to reduce hospital stay but not the other outcome measures. Various personality variables, such as denial, fear and aggressiveness were associated with the responses to these interventions. Less frightened patients benefited more from relaxation than did very frightened patients. *Wilson* speculated that the increased epinephrine levels were indicative of an active coping style. This would be consistent with *Frankenhaueser's* observations of positive correlations between epinephrine levels and the ability to cope with stressful experiences [74].

One other attempt to individualize treatment according to differences in personality style was reported by *Auerbach* [75]. Oral surgery patients were identified as having either an internal or external locus of control. Internal control subjects had an improved recovery from surgery when presented with specific information; whereas external control subjects did better when presented with general information prior to surgery.

Conclusions

There is well documented evidence that psychological and behavioral preparation prior to surgery can effect post-operative recovery. In almost all instances, except when patients are characterized by avoidance or denial defences predominantly, the outcome results have been positive. The effect of interventions have been most consistently positive in reducing length of hospitalization and post-operative pain, but a variety of other improvements in affect and physiologic stability have been shown. As others such as *Auerbach* have pointed out [76], in all but a handful of studies different intervention approaches have been combined, making it impossible to sort out the specific effects of information, psychotherapeutic relationship, relaxation training, or suggestion given either with or without hypnosis. Indeed it is not only likely that each has had an effect, but there may also be synergistic effects.

More recent investigations have begun to include measurements of personality differences between patients so that the nature of the intervention can be more specific and appropriate to the individual's coping style.

The reduction in length of hospitalization alone (clearly shown to result from pre-operative psychologic preparation) argues forcefully on a cost benefit basis for the inclusion of careful pre-operative preparation. The reduction in pain is also of major importance, and may well reduce future avoidance behavior or post-traumatic disorders, although these latter potential outcomes have not been investigated. It should be kept in mind that there are also a number of studies which have failed to demonstrate the efficacy of psychological intervention on these outcome measures. Moreover, it is extremely difficult in studies of this nature to control adequately for the subtle effects on behavior of experimenter and subject expectation.

A few points can be made about future strategies in this field. The evidence accumulated to date suggests that all patients undergoing surgery or certain difficult procedures be given the option of pre-operative psychological preparation. The preparation should emphasize what the patient will experience and when, and how to cope with it, i.e., how to move, or breathe, or relax. Rapidly evolving audiovisual capabilities and hospital televisions connected by cable to health education channels will routinely offer such preparation in the future. Patients could choose or not choose to watch (thereby protecting mechanisms of denial).

Finally, future studies should focus on outcome measures uniquely important to a particular operation and also on longer term rehabilitation outcome measures. An example of the former might be post-operative sexual functioning after prostatectomy. A study by *Zokar* et al. [77] has shown that the likelihood of this post-operative function is correlated with not only the level of pre-operative anxiety and general 'life satisfaction', but also whether the patient received a pre-operative explanation of what to expect from the surgery.

References

1   Price, D.B.; Thaler, M.; Mason, J.W.: Preoperative emotional states and adrenal cortical activity; studies on cardiac and pulmonary patients. Arch. Neurol. Psychiat. *77:* 646–656 (1957).

2   Czeisler, C.A.; Moore Ede, M.C.; Regestein, Q.R.; et al.: Episodic 24-hour cortisol secretory patterns in patients awaiting cardiac surgery. J. Clin. Endocrin. Metabol. *42:* 273–283 (1976).

3   Greene, W.; Conron, G.; Schalch, D.S.; et al.: Psychologic correlates of growth hormone and adrenal secretory responses of patients undergoing cardiac catheterization. Psychosom. Med. *32:* 599–614 (1970).

4   Barnes, C.M.; Kenny, F.M.; Thomas, C.; et al.: Measurement in management of anxiety in children for open heart surgery. Pediatrics *49:* 250–259 (1971).

5   Katz, J.; Weiner, H.; Gallagher, T.E.; et al.: Stress, distress, and ego defenses: psychoendocrine responses to impending breast tumor biopsy. Arch Gen. Psychiat. *23:* 131–142 (1970).

6   Wolff, C.T.; Hofer, M.A.; Mason, J.W.: Relationship between psychological defenses and mean urinary 17-hydroxycorticosteroid excretion rates. II Methodological and theoretical considerations. Psychosom. Med. *26:* 592–609 (1964).

7   Knight, R.B.; Atkins, A.; Eagle, C.J.; et al.: Psychological stress, ego defenses and cortisol production in children hospitalized for elective surgery. Psychosom. Med. *41:* 40–49 (1979).

8   Slade, M.S.; Simmons, R.K.; Yunis, E.; Greenberg, C.J.: Immunodepression after major surgery in normal patients. Surgery *78:* 363–372 (1975).

9   Janis, I.L.: Psychological Stress (Wiley, New York 1958).

10   Sime, A.M.: Relationship of pre-operative fear, type of coping and information received about surgery to recovery from surgery. J. Pers. Soc. Psychot. *34:* 716–724 (1976).

11   Jessner, L.; Blom, G.E.; Waldfogel, S.: Emotional implications of tonsillectomy and adenoidectomy on children. Psychoanal. Stud. Child 7: 126 (1952).

12   Eckenhoff, J.E.: Relationship of anesthesia to postoperative personality changes in children. Am. J. Dis. Child 86: 587 (1953).

13   Parker, J.B.: Psychiatric aspects of sterilization; in H.S. Abram, Psychological Aspects of Surgery, International Psychiatry Clinics, No. 4, pp. 105–113 (Little, Brown & Co. Boston, 1967).

14   Swanson, D.W.: Clinical psychiatric problems associated with general surgery; in H.S. Abram, Psychological Aspects of Surgery, International Psychiatry Clinics, No. 4, pp. 53–73, (Little, Brown & Co. Boston, 1967).

15   Rogers, M.P.; Liang, M.H.; Poss, R.; Cullen, K.: Adverse psychological sequelae associated with total joint replacement surgery. Gen. Hosp. Psychiat. 4: 155–158 (1982).

16   Cohen, F.; Lazarus, R.S.: Active coping processes, coping dispositions, and recovery from surgery. Psychosom. Med. 35: 375–389 (1973).

17   Wolfer, J.A.; Davis, C.E.: Assessment of Surgical patients Preoperative Emotional Conditions and Postoperative Welfare. Nursing Res. 19: 402–414 (1970).

18   Egbert, L.D.; Battit, G.E.; Turndorf, H.; Beecher, H.K.: The value of the preoperative visit by an anesthetist. JAMA 185: 553 (1963).

19   Egbert, L.D.; Battit, G.E.; Welch, C.E.; Barlett, M.K.: Reduction of postoperative pain by encouragement and instruction of patients. New Eng. J. Med. 270: 825 (1964).

20   Healy, K.M.: Does preoperative instruction make a difference? Am. J. Nursing 68: 62–67 (1968).

21   Johnson, J.E.; Rice, V.H.; Fuller, S.S.; Endress, M.P.: Sensory information, instruction in a coping strategy, and recovery from surgery. Nursing Res. Health 1: 4–17 (1978).

22   Lindeman, C.A.; Stetzer, S.L.: Effects of preoperative visits by operating room nurses. Nursing Res. 22: 4–16 (1973).

23   Lindeman, C.A.; Van Aernam, B.: Nursing intervention with the presurgical patients: the effects of structured and unstructured preoperative teaching. Nursing Res. 20: 319–332 (1971).

24   Surman, O.S.; Hackett, T.P.; Silverberg, E.L.; et al.: Usefulness of psychiatric intervention in patients undergoing cardiac surgery. Arch. Gen. Psychiat. 30: 830–835 (1974).

25   Archuleta, V.; Plummer, O.B.; Hopkins, D.K.: Administration model for patient education: A model for the project; in Boulder, project report (Western State Commission for Higher Education, June 1977).

26   Schmitt, F.E.; Wooldrige, P.J.: Psychological preparation of surgical patients. Nursing Res. 22: 108–116 (1973).

27   Langer, E.J.; Janis, I.L.; Wolfer, J.A.: Reduction of psychological stress in surgical patients. J. Exp. Soc. Psychol. 11: 155–163 (1975).

28   Fortin, F.; Kirouac, S.: A randomized controlled trial of preoperative patient education. Int. J. Nurs. Stud. 13: 83–96 (1976).

29   Flagherty, G.G.; Fitzpatrick, J.J.: Relaxation technique to increase comfort level of postoperative patients: a preliminary study. Nursing Res. 27: 352–355 (1978).

30   Mumford, E.; Schlesinger, H.J.; Glass, G.V.: The effects of psychological intervention on recovery from surgery and heart attacks: An analysis of the literature. Amer. J. Pub. Health 72: 141–151 (1982).

31   Levitan, S.J.; Kornfeld, D.S.: Clinical and cost benefits of liaison psychiatry. Am. J. Psychiat. 138: 790–793 (1981).

32   Kornfeld, D.S.; Heller, S.S.; Frank, K.A.; Moskowitz, R.: Personality and psychological factors in post-cardiotomy delirium. Arch. Gen. Psychiat. *31:* 249–253 (1974).

33   Blachy, P.H.; Starr, A.: Post-cardiotomy delirium. Am. J. Psychiat. *121:* 371–375 (1964).

34   Heller, S.S.; Frank, K.A.; Malm, J.R.; et al.: Psychiatric complications of open-heart surgery: a re-examination. New Eng. J. Med. *283:* 1015–1020 (1970).

35   Weisman, A.D.; Hackett, T.P.: Psychosis after eye surgery: establishment of specific doctor-patient relationship in prevention and treatment of black patch delirium. New Eng. J. Med. *258:* 1284–1289 (1958).

36   Millar, H.R.: Psychiatric morbidity in elderly surgical patients. Brit. J. Psychiat. *138:* 17–20 (1981).

37   Titchener, J.; Zwerling, I.; Gottschalk, L.; Levine, M.: Psychological reactions of the aged in surgery. Arch. Neurol. Psychiat. *79:* 63–73 (1958).

38   Sheppeard, H.; Cleak, D.K.; Ward, D.J.; O'Connor, B.T.: A review of early mortality and morbidity in elderly patients following Charnley total hip replacement. Arch. Orthoped. Traumat. Surg. *97:* 243–248 (1980).

39   Lazarus, H.R.; Hagens, J.H.: Prevention of psychosis following open-heart surgery. Am. J. Psychiat. *124:* 1190–1195 (1968).

40   Layne, O.L.; Yudofsky, S.C.: Postoperative psychosis in cardiotomy patients. New Eng. J. Med. *284:* 518–520 (1971).

41   Aiken, L.H.; Henrichs, T.F.: Systematic relaxation as a nursing intervention technique with open heart surgery patients. Nursing Res. *20:* 212–217 (1971).

42   Owens, J.F.; Hutelmyer, C.M.: The effect of preoperative intervention of delirium on cardiac surgical patients. Nursing Res. *31:* 60–62 (1982).

43   Johnson, J.E.: Effects of structuring patients' expectations on their reactions to threatening events. Nursing Res. *21:* 499–504 (1972).

44   Johnson, J.E.; Morrissey, J.F.; Leventhal, H.: Psychological preparation for an endoscope examination. Gastro-intest. Endosc. *19:* 180–182 (1973).

45   Corah, N.L.: Relaxation and musical programming as a means of reducing psychological stress during dental procedures. J. Am. Dent. Assoc. *103:* 232–234 (1981).

46   Nocella, J.: Training children to cope with dental treatment. J. Pediat. Psychol. *7:* 175–178 (1982).

47   Beck, N.C.; Siegel, L.J.: Preparation for childbirth and contemporary research on pain, anxiety, and stress reduction. A review and critique. Psychosom. Med. *42:* 429–447 (1980).

48   Finesilver, C.: Preparation of adult patients for cardiac catheterization and coronary cineangiography. Int. J. Nurs. Stud. *15:* 211–221 (1978).

49   Dumas, R.G.; Leonard, R.C.: The effect of nursing on the incidence of postoperative vomiting. Nursing Res. *12:* 12–15 (1963).

50   Felton, G.; Huss, K.; Payne, E.A.; et al.: Preoperative nursing intervention with the patient for surgery: outcomes of three alternative approaches. Int. J. Nurs. Stud. *13:* 83–96 (1976).

51   Bonilla, K.B.; Quigley, W.F.; Bowers, W.F.: Experiences with hypnosis on a surgical service. Milit. Med. *126:* 364–370 (1961).

52   Fortin, F.; Kirouac, S.: A randomized controlled trial of preoperative patient education. Int. J. Nurs. Stud. *13:* 11–24 (1976).

53   Treiger, P.; Tovarek, J.J.; Casciate, N.A.: Physiopsychologic treatment for postoperative urinary retention. Am. J. Surg. *80:* 195–197 (1950).

54   Florell, J.L.: Crisis intervention in orthopedic surgery, Doctoral dissertation. Dissertation abstracts international *32:* 3633B, microfilms no. 71–30, 799 (Northwestern Univ. 1971).

55   Ray, C.; Fitzgibbon, G.: Stress arousal and coping with surgery. Psychol. Med. *11:* 741–746 (1981).

56   Auerbach, S.M.: Trait-state anxiety and adjustment to surgery. J. Consult. Clin. Psychol. *40:* 264–271 (1973).

57   Langer, E.J.; Janis, I.L.; Wolfer, J.A.: Reduction of psychological stress in surgical patients. J. Exp. Soc. Psychol. *11:* 155–165 (1975).

58   Vernon, D.T.A.; Bailey, W.C.: The use of motion pictures in the psychological preparation of children for induction of anesthesia. Anesthesiology *40:* 68–72 (1974).

59   Cassell, S.; Paul, M.H.: The role of puppet therapy on the emotional responses of children hospitalized for cardiac catheterization. J. Peds. *71:* 233–239 (1967).

60   Mahaffy, P.R.: The effects of hospitalization on children admitted for tonsillectomy and adenoidectomy. Nursing Res. *14:* 12–19 (1965).

61   Danchin, N.; David, P.; Robert, P.; Bourassa, M.G.: Return to work after coronary surgery: Is there a need for a comprehensive rehabilitation program?; in Mathes, P.; Halhuber, J., Controversies in cardiac rehabilitation, pp. 81–83, (Springer-Verlag, New York 1982).

62   Naismith, L.D.; Robinson, J.F.; Shaw, G.B.; MacIntyre, M.M.: Psychological rehabilitation after myocardial infarction. Brit. Med. J. *1:* 439–446 (1979).

63   Staub, E.; Tursky, B.; Schwartz, G.E.: Self-control and predictability. Their effects on reactions to aversive stimulation. J. Pers. Soc. Psychol. *18:* 157–162 (1971).

64   Kolouch, F.T.: Hypnosis and surgical convalescence: a study of subjective factors in postoperative recovery. Am. J. Clin. Hypn. *7:* 120–129 (1964).

65   Doberneck, R.C.; Griffin, W.O. Jr.; Papermaster, A.A.; et al.: Hypnosis as an adjunct to surgical therapy. Surgery *46:* 299–304 (1959).

66   Gruen, W.: A successful application of systematic self-relaxation and self-suggestions about postoperative reactions in a case of cardiac surgery. Int. J. Clin. Exp. Hypn. *20:* 143–151 (1972).

67   Wilson, J.F.: Behavioral preparation for surgery benefit or harm? J. Behav. Med. *4:* 79–102 (1981).

68   Field, P.: Effects of tape recorded hypnotic preparation for surgery. Int. J. Clin. Hypn. *22:* 54–61 (1974).

69   Smith, L.S.: An investigation of pre- and post-surgical anxiety as a function of relaxation training. Doctoral dissertation (University of Southern Mississippi, Hattiesburg, 1974).

70   Andrew, J.M.: Recovery from surgery, with and without preparatory instruction, for three coping styles. J. Pers. Soc. Psychol. *15:* 223–226 (1970).

71   Delong, D.R.: Individual differences in patterns of anxiety arousal, stress-relevant information, and recovery from surgery. Unpublished doctoral dissertation (University of California, Los Angeles, 1970).

72   Shipley, R.H.; Butt, J.H.; Horowitz, E.A.; Farbry, J.E.: Preparation for a stressful medical procedure: effect of amount of stimulus pre-exposure and coping style. J. Consult. Clin. Psychol. *46:* 499–507 (1978).

73   Klos, D.; Cummings, M.; Joyce, J.; et al.: A comparison of two methods of delivering presurgical instructions. Patient Counselling and Health Education. First quarter: 6–13 (1980).

74   Frankenhaeuser, M.: Psychoneuroendocrine approaches to the study of emotion as related to stress and coping. Nebr. Symp. Motiv. *26:* 123–161 (1978).

75   Auerbach, S.M.; Kendall, P.C.; Cuttler, H.F.; Levitt, N.R.: Anxiety, locus of control, type

of preparatory information, and adjustment to dental surgery. J. Consult. Clin. Psychol. *44:* 809–818 (1976).

76   Auerbach, S.M.; Kulmann, P.R.: Crisis intervention: a review of outcome research. Psychol. Bull. *84:* 1189–1217 (1977).

77   Zohar, J.; Meiraz, D.; Mooz, B.; Durst, N.: Factors influencing sexual activity after prostatectomy: A prospective study. J. Urol. *116:* 332–334 (1976).

Malcolm Rogers, MD, Harvard Medical School, Brigham and Women's Hospital, Boston, MA 02115 (USA)

Adv. psychosom. Med., vol. 15, pp. 51–68 (Karger, Basel 1986)

Post-Operative Delirium

Larry Tune, Marshal F. Folstein

The Johns Hopkins University School of Medicine and Director, Dementia Research Clinic; Departments of Medicine and Psychiatry and Behavioral Science, Division of General Hospital Psychiatry, Johns Hopkins Hospital, Baltimore, Md., USA

This chapter reviews the syndrome of delirium from a phenomenological perspective, and then in this context, focuses on the subject of post-operative delirium. Disturbance of consciousness, the defining feature of delirium, is a phenomenon everyone experiences under certain circumstances, for example after sleep, during intoxication, and during recovery from general anesthesia. Mild symptoms of delirium are common during any systemic illness, and are experienced as lethargy, distractability, and a decrease in normal alertness. More profound delirium occurs in seriously ill patients, and can cause dramatic symptoms, including vivid hallucinations, delusions and mood swings, all of which can seriously interfere with the hospital care.

Although these symptoms are potentially reversible and are not a sign of impending chronic mental illness or dementia, delirium is often associated with a fatal outcome. In one study, 25% of patients with delirium admitted to a general medical ward died during the index admission [1]. Even when not fatal, it can be the cause of prolonged disability and lengthened hospital stay. For example, the morbidity resulting from a delirious state after a simple herniorraphy may delay early mobilization of the patient, thereby contributing to the development of pneumonia, pulmonary embolus or sepsis secondary to infected bed sores.

If serious complications are to be avoided, swift recognition of delirium is critical so that the underlying metabolic cause can be indentified and treated, and the distressing psychological symptoms brought to an end. Recognition of early symptoms of delirium is of particular importance following outpatient surgery since the patient leaves hospital observation and care within hours of the procedure.

Deterrents to Research in Delirium

In spite of the apparent importance of delirium in surgical and medical practice, its mechanism is unknown. There are many aspects of delirious patients which perpetuate our ignorance. First, many of these patients are severely medically ill, and therefore difficult to study. Second, the delirious state often resolves quickly and completely with treatment of the underlying cause, rendering clinical trials or studies of the pathophysiology difficult to plan and carry out. Third, when clinical research has been attempted, lack of: standard definitions, standard criteria or standardized means of measuring the delirious state has resulted in much confusion. As a result, existing studies use different terminology, making growth of knowledge through comparibility of studies impossible.

One area of confusion, then, concerns terminology: between those states identified as understandable reactions to the stress of surgery, for example, post-operative anxiety, depression, and agitation and post-operative delirium.

The second area of confusion concerns diagnosis, especially regarding those subtypes initially described by *Bonhoeffer* [3]. Presently, the Diagnostic and Statistical Manual of the American Psychiatric Association (DSM-III) [4] considers delirium to be a simple category which encompasses *Bonhoeffer's* subtypes [3]. However, neurological practice now generally employs the term 'delirium' to refer to the agitated, tremulous, hallucinatory state, such as that which occurs during delirium tremens, and uses the term 'acute confusional state' to refer to the drowsy, somnolant state which accompanies severe metabolic disorders such as hepatic insufficiency [2, 5]. A survey of 106 cases by *Wolff and Curran* in 1935 [6] confirmed *Bonhoeffer's* concept of a simple reaction type. They postulated that delirium is a syndrome characterized by a disturbance of consciousness and cognitive impairment, which, regardless of cause, is often accompained by a variety of other psychiatric symptoms.

Romano and Engel in the 1940's provided the first pathological correlation of delirium when they studied the EEG in delirious patients and found a diffusely slow record to be characteristic [7]. *Moruzzia and Magoun* linked

Table I. Diagnostic criteria for delirium (DSM-111)

A. Clouding of consciousness (reduced clarity of awareness of the environment), with reduced capacity to shift, focus, and sustain attention to environmental stimuli.

B. At least two of the following:
    (1) Perceptual disturbance: misinterpretations, illusions, or hallucinations
    (2) Speech that is at times incoherent
    (3) Disturbance of sleep-wakefulness cycle, with insomnia or daytime drowsiness
    (4) Increased or decreased psychomotor activity

C. Disorientation and memory impairment (if testable)

D. Clinical features that develop over a short period of time (usually hours to days) and tend to fluctuate over the course of a day

E. Evidence, from the history, physical examination, or laboratory tests, of a specific organic factor judged to be etiologically related to the disturbance

---

a change in the consciousness of animals with a slow wave EEG frequencies and lesions strategically placed in the reticular activating system [8]. More recently, *Shute and Lewis* identified acetylcholine as a neurotransmitter of this system [9]. Although all authors do not agree with the generality of these findings, most would agree that delirium is a syndrome characterized by a disturbance of consciousness, and that its cognitive sequelae, such as disturbances of memory and attention, usually accompanied by a slow EEG frequency, can also be seen following anesthesia or intoxications with agents that interfere with the cholinergic function of the reticular system or its connections.

Diagnostic Criteria for Delirium

Recently, criteria have been developed in the DSM-III [4] for the standardized diagnosis of delirium. These are seen in table I. Although these criteria do encompass the definition of delirium, the elimination of 'disturbance of consciousness' as a central feature or as a central criterion, may be an error. Equating 'attention' with 'consciousness' is plausible, but attention is altered in other, very different, clinical states, such as depression, mania or dementia, in which there is no clouding of consciousness.

The criteria for a clear case of delirium, we maintain, also includes some degree of cognitive impairment, especially attentional deficits (even though the specific term 'cognitive impairment' is not contained in the DSM-III criteria). The rapid onset, variability, and fluctuation of mental status are accessory rather than fundamental clinical features, thus not necessary for the diagnosis of delirium itself.

We find it clinically useful to subclassify delirium into two types: the vigilant type, as exemplified by delirium tremens, and the somnolant type, exemplified by most other metabolic disorders. A given patient can shift from a somnolant to a vigilant state during the same episode of delirious illness. Thus, the subtypes are not mutually exclusive. The basis for this classification is that the EEG of the somnolant type is often slower in its underlying frequencies than the vigilant type [1, 7, 10].

The determination of whether a given clinical state meets any set of diagnostic criteria depends on close observation of the patient, and the measurement and recording of signs and symptoms, preferably with the use of modern, standardized procedures. Such measurements can be made using the clinical method, i.e. while taking a history and doing a physical examination, or with structured psychological tests. However, in many cases of delirium, refined measurements are not possible because the patient is too disturbed to cooperate and the physical setting is unsuitable. Nevertheless, there are acceptable ways of measuring the level of consciousness, attention, and overall cognitive state of delirious patients so that these measurements can be matched against the criteria necessary for diagnosis.

Level of consciousness is best assessed by the examiner according to his/her observations of the patient's alertness and accessibility during a brief conversation or during the cognitive examination. The examiner's impression can then be recorded on an analogue scale. The reliability of this method, even in the hands of inexperienced medical students, is adequate, and ratings of alertness on analogue scales correlate significantly with the clinical ratings of EEG abnormalities as shown in table II [11].

Diagnostic Aids

Although disturbances of attention are prominent features of delirium, few methods for measuring attention are suitable for administration at the bedside. Portable devices are available for the measurement of signal detection and vigilance [12]. The measurement of perception time with the hand-held tachistoscope is a valid and sensitive method for the detection of delirium, but detects many false-positive cases and, therefore, must be used

Table II. Validity of measures of consciousness and cognition in delirium

Assessment	Measures			
	Analogue	Perception Time	Mini-mental State exam	EEG
	r	r	r	r
Consciousness by Alertness Analogue	–	0.6***	0.5***	0.6**
Attention by Perception time	0.6**	–	0.7**	0.6**
Cognitive Impairment by Mini-mental state exam	0.5*	0.7**	–	0.7***

* = 0.01.   ** = 0.005.   *** = 0.0005.

The cardinal features of delirium can be validly assessed by the clinical rating of consciousness, the measurement of perception, and cognitive screening with the MMS examination.

as a first stage screening procedure only. The reliability and validity of the tachistoscope as a measure of delirium is summarized in table II.

Most delirious patients suffer from moderate cognitive impairment which can be manifested by: disorientation, memory loss, difficulty with concentration, disturbance of attention, and difficulty with complex learned motor movements like handwriting [13]. There are several useful screening instruments for cognitive impairment which can be administered at the bedside by clinicians and technicians. The Mini-Mental State Examination is one such cognitive screening procedure which is of established reliability and validity [14]. Its specificity and sensitivity have been determined in general medical populations with delirium and dementia and are adequate for screening purposes [1]. However, in our series of delirious patients, approximately 30% of cases scored above the usual 'cut off' point of 23 on the Mini-Mental State Examination but still had scores which were less than optimal, since their scores increased as the delirium cleared.

Table III. Mini-mental state examination

Patient: _____

Examiner: _____

Date: _____

Maximum Score	Score	
		Orientation
5	( )	What is the: (year) (season) (date) (day) (month)?
5	( )	Where are we: (state) (country) (town) (hospital) (floor)?
		Registration
3	( )	Name 3 objects: 1 second to say each. Then ask patient all 3 after you have said them. Give 1 point for each correct answer. Then repeat them until he learns all 3. Count trials and record. _____ trials.
		Attention and calculation
5	( )	Serial 7's. 1 point for each correct. Stop after 5 answers. Alternatively spell "world" backwards.
		Recall
3	( )	Ask for the 3 objects repeated above. Give 1 point for each correct.
		Language
9	( )	Name a pencil, and watch (2 points).
		Repeat the following: "No ifs, ands, or buts." (1 point)
		Follow a 3-stage command:
		"Take a paper in your right hand, fold it in half and put it on the floor." (3 points)
		Read and obey the following:
		"Close your eyes " (1 point)
		Write a sentence. (1 point)
		Copy design. (1 point)
_____		Total score

Assess level of consciousness long a continuum

Alert	Drowsy	Stupor	Coma

The Mini-Mental State Examination (table III) is a 30-point examination which assesses orientation to time and place; registration of 3 objects; attention, concentration and calculation as assessed by the serial 7's task; and then the recall of the 3 objects. The second portion of the examination screens the patient's capacity to name simple objects, repeat, understand a command, read, write, and copy a design. Ninety-five percent of the population

Table IV. Abnormal mental phenomena in delirium

Phenomena	Diagnostic groups		
	hepatic encephalopathy, %	delirium tremens, %	other, %
Hallucinations	62	76	63
Delusions	24	41	63
Depression	48	65	50
Anxiety	29	59	37

Dramatic disruptive and distressing psychiatric symptoms are frequent in delirium caused by liver failure, alcohol withdrawal, and other causes (data collected by Dr. U. Niaz).

of a sample of 3,841 persons living at home in Baltimore scored higher than 23 points on this examination. The sensitivity and specificity for detecting delirium and dementia is between 80–90%, depending on the cutting score chosen [11].

Non-Cognitive Symptoms

Cognitive symptoms are not the only symptoms in delirium. Additional symptoms can include abnormal phenomena such as hallucinations, abnormal goal-directed behaviors such as non-compliance, and abnormal motor signs including tremor, difficulty walking, and autonomic instability including tachycardia [2, 3, 5, 6, 13, 15–17]. The abnormal phenomena that occur in delirium are some of the most dramatic seen in medicine.

Hallucinations are often present [see table XV; ref. 6], especially visual hallucinations. They can range from pleasant visions of colored balloons to frightening visions of threatening visitors with distorted shapes. Hallucinations and illusions are, to a certain extent, responsive to environmental stimulation and tend to become worse when natural lighting becomes dim. This may contribute to the increased frequency of these phenomena in the evening – the 'sundowning' phenomena.

Visual hallucinations and illusions that occur in delirium sometimes give rise to delusions. Patients also respond to hallucinations with anxiety and depression (table IV).

Hallucinations and delusions of the delirious patient can be compared to a dream-like state: like the dream state, the effects of these experiences can extend beyond the actual episode of illness. Fortunately, delirium is usually associated with amnesia for events that occur during the delirious period. It is most common for these experiences to be completely forgotten.

Abnormal mood states, including depression and anxiety even leading to a sense of hopelessness and despair, can occur during delirium with or without relation to hallucinations and delusions. The depressed mood of the delirious patient can cause suicidal thoughts and behavior as well as an unrealistically pessimistic assessment of the patient's circumstances. It is important to recognize that the hopeless mood which occasionally accompanies delirium is a symptom related to the underlying medical disorder. The patient's attitude toward self and future will be modified if the delirium can be relieved even though the basis for medical prognosis remains the same. For this reason, a patient's request for the termination of treatment during a delirious episode in the course of a serious illness must be assessed in the context of the other features of the patient's mental state.

The combination of cognitive impairment, plus abnormal perceptions, beliefs and moods can lead to a variety of abnormal behaviors which are often interpreted as willful or even hostile. Thus, the delirious patient, because of the accompanying inability to understand, remember or attend, is often unable to comply with requests for cooperation with complex testing, such as pulmonary function testing or x-rays requiring relative motionlessness. Even drinking fluids on schedule can become impossible in the face of the delirium. During delirium, the patient's compliance will be increased if he/she can be sufficiently stimulated to attend to instructions. Other significant behaviors that can accompany the mood disturbance are suicidal behavior and combativeness.

Sleeping is typically abnormal in delirium, with the patient apparently striving for sleep but often awakening after a short time. The onset of a normal period of sleep often marks the end of the delirious episode.

Abnormal motor signs of almost every description can occur in delirious patients. There is ataxia, tremor, myoclonus, asterixis and bradykinesia. Finally delirious patients often have clear abnormalities of autonomic motor function including tachycardia and diapheresis.

Differential Diagnosis

Diagnostic errors are common. A frequent error is to attribute the patient's behavior to a 'functional psychiatric illness'. The language of the patient is attributed to 'schizophrenic word salad'; the apathy, to 'depression'; or the elated state experienced by the hypervigilant patient, to 'mania'. The label of 'functional psychiatric illness' can have fatal consequences for the patient with delirium, since what is often missed is acute infection, toxicity from medication or other potentially reversible states. A second error, as noted by *Mesulam and Geshwind* [2] is to diagnose an 'untreatable neurological disorder'. In this case, delirious patients are given the label of 'stroke' or 'senile dementia'.

These errors can be avoided by recognizing that the differential diagnosis in delirium has two steps: [1] the distinction of delirium from other psychiatric disorders and [2] the attribution of the delirium to a specific pathology. The key to the first step in establishing the diagnosis of delirium is to perform a mental status examination. This comment may seem obvious, but delirious patients are often given the label of 'hysteria' or 'schizophrenia' because the mental status of the patient was not taken into account. By identifying the alteration in the level of consciousness, the inaccessibility, the severe disturbance in thinking (including disturbances of attention, memory and orientation), and the disruption in the sleep/wake cycle, symptoms more specific to the diagnosis of delirium are recognized. The EEG can be helpful in identifying the delirious patient. Bilateral diffuse slowing of the EEG below 8–9 per second is usually found in all deliria, with the exception of delirum tremens. This can help in distinguishing delirium from hysteria and schizophrenia [2, 18].

Delirium is also sometimes misdiagnosed as dementia. The important, and obvious, distinction between the two conditions is that in delirium there is always some alteration in the level of consciousness, whereas the demented patient is cognitively impaired even when fully alert.

Post-Operative Delirium

Estimates of the incidence of post-operative delirium vary considerably from author to author. *Kelly* [19] has calculated the incidence of 'post-operative psychosis' as 1 per 400 cases of gynecological surgery. This estimate may be methodologically flawed, since it was used in a retrospective study of what appeared to be patients with functional psychotic illness. The nature of the gynecological surgery and the younger age of the patients clearly make this a special population. In a general surgical population, *Titchener* et al. [20] found 7.8 cases per 100, and *Tufo* et al. [21] found a prevalence of 24% of acute confusional state following open heart surgery.

Because of these varying reports, recent interest in the field has focused on variables likely to cause delirium. The nature of the surgery, age of patient, duration of surgery, medication history, and a variety of other factors may be important factors in the development of delirious states. The causes of delirium can be classified into predisposing pre-operative factors and precipitating post-operative factors.

Etiological Factors in the Pre-Operative Period

Table V provides a list of etiological factors in the pre-operative and post-operative periods leading to delirium.

Age

Age-related psychological, biochemical and anatomical changes increase the risk for post-operative delirium. The older patient possesses less ability to process information, to attend to tasks and to 'cope' with new stressful situations than the younger patient [22]. Electrophysiologically, the EEG slows with age, with slowing over the temporal areas, decreased alpha activity and altered reactivity to physiological stimuli. These changes resemble those occurring in delirious states. Changes in anatomy that occur with age may very well contribute to increased susceptibility to delirious states.

Alcohol Addiction

Addiction to alcohol, or possibly other drugs of abuse, increase risk of delirium [2, 10]. Before an operation, a patient may minimize or deny a history of drug abuse or dependency. Lack of appropriate pharmacologic treatment may lead to a withdrawal state in the immediate post-operative period, since typically, drug withdrawal occurs between 12 and 48 hours after cessation of the drug. Delirium tremens which, when untreated, is associated with

Table V. Factors associated with post-operative delirium

Factors originating in the pre-operative period	Factors originating intra-operatively or in the post-operative period
Increasing age (over 50) ? Psychiatric illness (psychosis, personality disorder)	Medications and drug combinations, esp. anticholinergics
Pre-operative factors causing special vulnerabilities	Sleep deprivation, sensory deprivation, and immobilization, low cardiac output post-operatively
Pre-operative dementia Susceptibility to toxins and metabolic abnormalities	Cerebrovascular accidents Length of time under anesthesia (8 + hours, 4 + hours bypass time)
Acute intermittent porphyria Drug sensitivities	Operative hypotension, hypercapnia, hypoxia, hypovolemia
Chronic renal disease Electrolyte abnormality Uremia Anemia Dialysis dysequilibrium	Choice of anesthetic Type of surgery (greater incidence with eye ops/complex surgeries) ? SICU environment
Neoplasm Metastasis Disseminated intravascular coagulopathy Nonbacterial endocarditis	Post-operative electrolyte abnormality, acid-base disturbances, anemia, hypoxia, abnormal PCO_2 hypoglycemia, uremia, hyperammonemia, endocrinopathies
Neurosyphillis Jarisch-Herxheimer reaction	Fever and infection
Addiction Withdrawal Thiamine deficiency	Cardiac, pulmonary, or abdominal complications
Traumatic injury Concussion Contusion Subdural hematoma Fat embolism	
Seizure disorders Postictal confusion	

15% mortality [10], is perhaps the most dramatic and readily identified of the delirious states.

Less commonly appreciated in the alcoholic patient is thiamine deficiency. The administration of intravenous glucose pre-operatively to patients with compensated or borderline nutritional status may lead to a serious or possibly fatal post-operative delirious state. In such instances, the typical post-operative syndrome is Wernicke-Korsakoff's psychosis. Clinical symptoms are nystagmus, ophthalmoplegia, ataxia, and a delirious state which often resolves to an amnestic syndrome. This syndrome is often not detected in the immediate post-operative period, since delirious patients are difficult to examine for subtle neurological signs.

Another etiology of delirium in the post-operative alcoholic patient is chronic subdural hematoma. These may be difficult to diagnose in substance abusing patients. However the presence of lateralizing neurological signs should raise the clinician's index of suspicion.

Post-Traumatic Patient

Acute trauma, brain concussion, contusions, subdural hematoma, or fat embolism, may be an important etiological factor in the development of post-operative delirium. As a result of acute blood loss, airway obstruction or the administration of medications, the trauma patient is particularly susceptible to the development of a delirious state in the first three days after admission. Of note, these first three days are likely to be the greatest 'at risk' for the development of an expanding subdural hematoma or fat embolism [23].

Seizure Disorder

Seizure disorders may cause delirium in post-operative patients. In the setting of acute stress, acute changes in homeostasis and acute changes in medication regimen, these patients are at greater risk of increased seizure activity [2]. Seizure-induced delirium may rarely last for up to several days post-ictally.

Etiological Factors in the Operative and Post-Operative Period

Anoxia

Table V [adopted from 2] provides a list of important factors in the intra- and post-operative periods that may contribute to the development of post-operative delirium. Of particular importance in the intra-operative period are the consequences of anoxia. These may result from hypotension, hypoxia, hyponatremia or anesthesia itself (e.g. nitrous oxide narcosis). In individuals undergoing open heart surgery, or elderly patients, the risk of transient or permanent sequelae from anoxia is serious [21, 24].

In patients dying while delirious in the post-operative period, neuropathological findings may reveal focal anoxic changes or infarction.

Toxic, Metabolic Abnormalities

Most post-operative delirious states are attributed to toxic or metabolic insults, including dehydration, anemia, hypoxia, acid-base imbalance, hypocarbia, hypercarbia, hypoglycemia, hyperosmolarity, hypotension, uremia, hyperammonemia, and endocrinopathies. These metabolic abnormalities all produce the same symptoms – delirium. Only laboratory tests will reveal the distinctions between them. Patients with severe organ disease, elderly patients, and patients with pre-existing metabolic abnormalities are a great risk for delirium in response to one of these insults [2].

Fever and Infection

Fever and infections which can cause delirium are not confined to infections of the nervous system. Pneumonia and urinary tract infections are often recognized as causes of confusional states, particularly in the elderly. It is our own experience that the symptoms of delirium occur very early in the course of pneumonia and can precede changes in the chest x-ray.

Drugs

Many drugs and drug combinations have been associated with acute onset of delirious states. In particular, psychoactive drugs, drugs with anticholinergic properties (for example, anti-Parkinsonian agents) and commonly prescribed cardiac medications (e.g. digoxin, procainamide, lidocaine) have been associated with acute confusional states [18, 25, 26]. In one study, 60 patients with post-operative confusion were compared to 57 age-matched controls. Those patients who developed post-operative delirium received significantly more drugs. In our own studies [27] of post-cardiotomy delirium, significant change in mental status examination was associated with increasingly elevated serum anticholinergic drug level (as determined by radioreceptor assay). Figure 1 gives the results of that study.

Twenty-nine patients who had undergone open heart surgery were evaluated pre- and 24 hours post-operatively for change in mental status. Each patient was evaluated with the Mini-Mental State Examination Score

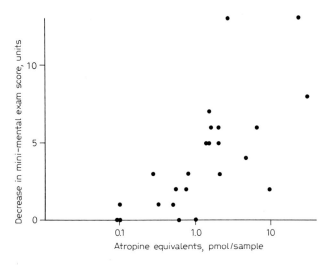

Fig. 1. Results of post-cardiotomy study. Change in clinical state in relation to serum anti-cholinergic levels in 18 patients who underwent 24 post-cardiotomy assessments. Clinical state is expressed as the change in mini-mental state examscore between pre-cardiotomy and post-cardiotomy ratings. The correlation coefficient was $r = -0.83$; $n = 24$; $p < 0.001$. Taken from: Tune, et al., 'Association of postoperative delirium with raised serum levels of anticholinergic drugs', The Lancet, pp. 652, Sept. 1981.

[14]. A significant change in mental status was defined as a decrease in the Mini-Mental State Exmination Score of 2 or more points. Figure 1 illustrates that, as Mental Status Examination Score declined, serum anticholinergic drug level increased. When these patients were evaluated according to the method of *Sommers* [28] for medication regimens known to be allied with confusional states, patients who developed post-operative delirium were found to have higher numbers of these medications.

In reviewing a case history it is often difficult to establish whether psychoactive drugs are causing the delirium or whether they have been prescribed after the symptoms of delirium have appeared. The institution of any psychoactive drug therapy, including sedatives and analgesics, should be accompanied by a mental state examination. According to *Lipowski* [18], drugs with anticholinergic properties are the most common cause of delirium among the elderly and have been implicated in numerous studies as etiologically important in the genesis of post-operative delirium. Thus, drug combinations, particularly those with anticholinergic properties, are to be avoided if possible.

Further evidence of the role of anticholinergic drugs in the genesis of delirium is found in a related study [29]. Twenty patients undergoing electro-convulsive therapy (ECT) for affective disorder were evaluated pre- and 1 hour post-ETC, assessing Mini-Mental State Examinations and serum anti-cholinergic levels. Since cognitive recovery from ECT can vary, the hypo-thesis was that delayed recovery from ECT was related to anticholinergic in-toxication. In this population, atropine, methohexital, and succinylcholine were all administered prior to ECT. Eight of 12 patients with elevated anti-cholinergic levels (greater than 15 ng/ml atropine equivalents) showed sig-nificant cognitive impairments (defined operationally as a decline of 2 or more points in Mini-Mental State Examinations where post and pre-ECT MMSE's were compared). By contrast only 1 of 8 patients with lower levels (less than 15 ng/ml atropine equivalents) showed such a decline. This study may serve as a model for the confusional states and emerging delirium asso-ciated with surgical procedures performed with brief anesthesia adminis-tered intravenously.

Physical Environment

Attempts to identify aspects of psychological import in the patient's environment which contribute to the development of post-operative delirium have led to the identification of the 'ICU syndrome'. It has been postulated that the stressful 'high tech' environment of intensive care units may have a role in the pathophysiology of these clinical syndromes [2, 7, 30–33]. One interpretation of these studies is that many patients are quietly delirious and unrecognized, but that a strange and stressful environment will produce dra-matic symptoms that are then recognized as delirium. Attempts to diminish the stress, by providing an empathic environment that facilitates the patient's reorientation and diminishes the level of stress and concern, have a common-sense appeal. In some studies this approach has been associated with a decreased incidence of delirious states [32].

Treatment

Treatment of post-operative delirium is based on rational, empirical, and empathic methods. Rational methods require a knowledge of precipitat-ing features, which are usually drug intoxication or metabolic imbalance due to major organ failure. Reduction of all medication is often a helpful first step in treatment. Cognitive monitoring of patients during hospitalization or when medications are being changed in elderly patients, will provide a useful marker to document improvement after appropriate treatment, or deterioration, as when patients are suffering from side effects of drugs.

Empirical treatments can be categorized as environmental and pharmacological. An optimal environment for the delirious patient requires close supervision that can be provided by many individuals. Ingenuity is often required to construct a schedule of visits from medical staff, occupational and physical therapists, nurses, volunteers, social workers and family.

The cooperation of the family can be better elicited by a careful explanation of the patient's state. Family members should be instructed to reorient the patient and maintain his/her contact with the present situation. Appropriate regulation of room lighting and the use of calendars are helpful in maintaining the patient's orientation. When persons enter the room, they should introduce themselves to the patient by stating their name and purpose. Any needed diagnostic or therapeutic procedure should be carefully and simply explained to the patient. Because delirious patients suffer from attention and memory impairment, such introductions and explanations must be made repeatedly.

Pharmacological treatments include benzodiazepines for the management of alcohol withdrawal; dopaminergic blockage with haloperidol (1 mg–2 mg three times a day orally or intramuscularly) for delirium of nonspecific cause with agitation; and anticholinesterase agents, such as physostigmine, for anticholinergically-induced delirium. Although the use of these drugs forms the basis for clinical practice, adequate clinical trials that specify dosage and duration of treatment are needed. There is little evidence currently available that pharmacological interventions alter the duration of the delirious state, but clinical practice suggests that they are of great utility for patient management.

Although delirious patients are cognitively impaired, their adequate treatment requires the empathy of physicians and hospital staff. Empathy with the delirious patient begins with inquiring about, and understanding, the patient's current fears, delusions, and hallucinations. Next follows clarification and reassurance concerning the specifics of fears and/or perplexing experiences. If the underlying medical condition is in fact reversible, reassurance is appropriate. If the medical condition is not reversible, the delirious stage should serve as an indication to maintain regular contacts with the patient. Terminal medical illness is sometimes seen by physicians as a sign of their failure and can result in a decrease in the frequency of visits to the patient. Physicians and staff visiting can be encouraged by helping them to see the visit to the dying patient as an opportunity to relieve suffering.

Empathy is also needed to appreciate the fears of the delirious patient's family members, who often fear that the delirium represents the onset of a permanent psychosis. The physician managing the delirious patient must also be able to empathize with the hospital staff in direct contact with the patient. The day-to-day caregivers are often frustrated by the patient's incapacity to cooperate with diagnostic and therapeutic procedures. Often a staff discussion of the manifestations of delirium can smooth the patient's hospital course.

The prevention of delirium comes with the recognition of predisposing features, cautious use of all medications, and the frequent monitoring of patient's state of consciousness, cognitive state, and sleep and dream pattern. Detection of the earliest signs of delirium enables the prevention of the secondary complications that occur when the patient becomes more seriously impaired in the capacity to appreciate his/her surroundings.

References

1   Rabins, P.V.; Folstein, M.F.: Delirium and dementia: Diagnostic criteria and fatality rates. Brit. J. Psychiat. *140:* 149–153 (1982).

2   Mesulam, M.M.; Geschwind, N.: Disordered mental states in the post-operative period. Urol. Clin. Na. *3:* 199–215 (1976).

3   Bonhoeffer, K.: Die Psychosen im Gefolge von akuten Infektionen und Allgemeiner-krankungen; in Aschaffenberg, G.L. ed., Handbuch der Psychiatrie, Spez. Teil. 3, pp. 1–60 (Leipzig, Denticke, 1912).

4   American Psychiatric Association, Diagnostic and statistical Manual of mental disorders (DSM-111) (APA, Washington, D.C., 1980).

5   Adams, R.D.; Victor, M.: Delirium and other confusional states; in Wintrobe, M.M.; Thorn, G.W.; Adams, R.D.; et al. (eds), Principles of internal medicine (McGraw Hill Book Co., New York 1974).

6   Wolff, H.S.; Curran, D.: Nature of delirium and allied states. The dysergastic reaction. Archs Neurol. Psychiat. *33:* 1175–1215 (1935).

7   Engel, G.L.; Romano, J.: Delirium. A syndrome of cerebral insufficiency. J. Chron. Dis. *9:* 260–277 (1959).

8   Moruzzi, G.; Magoun, H.: Brainstem reticular formation and actuation of the EEG. Electroencephalogr. Clin. Neurophys. *1:* 455–473 (1949).

9   Shute, C.C.D.; Lewis, P.R.: The ascending cholinergic reticular system: neocortical, olfactory, and subcortical projections. Brain *90:* 497–540 (1967).

10   Victor, M.; Adams, R.D.: The effect of alcohol upon the nervous system. Res. Publ. Assoc. Res. Nerv. Ment. Dis. *32:* 526–573 (1953).

11   Anthony, J.C.; LeResche, L.; Niaz, U.; VonKorff, M.F.; Folstein, M.F.: Limits of the

'Mini-Mental State' as a screening test for dementia and delirium among hospital patients. Psychol. Med. *12:* 397–408 (1982).

12 Pauker, N.; Folstein, M.F.; Moran, T.: The clinical utility of the hand-held tachistoscope. J. Nerv. Ment. Dis. *166:* 126–129 (1978).

13 Chedru, F.; Geschwind, N.: Disorders of higher cortical functions in acute confusional states. Cortex *8:* 395–411 (1972).

14 Folstein, M.F.; Folstein, S.E.; McHugh, P.R.: 'Mini-Mental State'. A practical method for grading the cognitive state of patients for the clinician. J. Psychiat. Res. *12*(3): 189–198 (1975).

15 Lipowski, Z.J.: Delirium, clouding of consciousness and confusion. J. Nerv. Ment. Dis. *145:* 227–255 (1967).

16 Cohen, S.: The toxic psychoses and allied states. Am. J. Med. *15:* 813–828 (1953).

17 Ludwig, A.M.: Altered states of consciousness. Archs Gen. Psychiat. *15:* 225–234 (1966).

18 Lipowski, Z.J.: Delirium: Acute brain failure in man. (C.C. Thomas, New York 1980).

19 Kelly, H.A.: Postoperative psychoses. Am. J. Obstet. Gynec. *59:* 1035–1037 (1909).

20 Titchener, J.L.; Zwerling, I.; Gottschalk, L.; et al.: Psychosis in surgical patients. Surg. Gynec. Obstet. *102:* 59–65 (1956).

21 Tufo, H.M.; Ostfeld, A.M.; Shekelle, R.: Central nervous system dysfunction following open-heart surgery. J. Am. med. Ass. *212:* 1333–1340 (1970).

22 Blass, J.; Plum, F.: Metabolic encephalopathies in older adult; in Plum, F. ed. The neurology of aging, pp. 189–219 (Davis, New York 1982).

23 Dines, D.E.; Burgher, L.W.; Okazaki, H.: The clinical and pathological correlation of fat embolism syndrome. Mayo Clinic Proc. *50:* 407–411 (1975).

24 Bedford, P.D.: Adverse cerebral effects of anaesthesia on old people. Lancet *2:* 259–263 (1955).

25 Ketchum, J.S.; Sidell, F.R.; Crowell, E.B.; Aghajanian, G.K.; Hayes, A.H.: Atropine, scopalamine, and Ditran: Comparative pharmacology and antagonists in man. Psychopharmacol. *28:* 121–145 (1943).

26 Morse, R.M.; Litin, E.M.: Postoperative delirium: a study of etiological factors. Am. J. Psychiat. *126:* 388–395 (1969)

27 Tune, L.; Holland, A.; Folstein, M.; Damlouji, N.; Gardner, T.; Coyle, J.T.: Association of post-operative delirium with raised level anticholinergic drugs. Lancet *11:* 650–652 (1981).

28 Summers, W.R.: A clinical method of estimating risk of drug-induced delirium. Life Sci. *22:* 1511–1516 (1978).

29 Mondimore, F.; Damlouji, N.; Folstein, M.F.; Tune, L.: Post-ECT confusional states associated with elevated anticholinergic levels. Am. J. Psychiat. *140:* 930–931 (1983).

30 Morris, G.O.; Singer, M.P.: Sleep deprivation: The content of consciousness. J. Nerv. Ment. Dis. *143:* 291–3045 (1966).

31 Scott, J.: Postoperative psychosis in the aged. Am. J. Surg. *100:* 38–42 (1960).

32 Taylor, D.E.M.: Problems of patients in an intensive care unit: The aetiology and prevention of the intensive care syndrome. Int. J. Nursing Stud. *8:* 47–59 (1971).

33 Dubin, W.R.; Field, H.L.; Gastfriend, D.R.: Postcardiotomy Delirium: A critical review. J. Thorac. Cardiovasc. Surg. *77:* 586–594 (1979).

Larry Tune, MD, Director, Dementia Research Clinic, Johns Hopkins University School of Medicine, Baltimore, MD 21205 (USA)

Adv. psychosom. Med., vol. 15, pp. 69–83 (Karger, Basel 1986)

Surgery in Infants, Children, and Adolescents

H. Paul Gabriel

Professor of Clinical Psychiatry, Department of Psychiatry, New York University
Medical Center, and Associate Attending, New York University Hospital, and Bellevue
Hospital, New York, N.Y., USA

During the past forty years, staggering advances in medicine have made possible operations of increasing technical complexity [8, 9]. Over the same period, psychiatrists have acquired greater understanding of the special needs of children and young people who must undergo the particular stresses of major surgery. This chapter will delineate those issues of most concern to the medical specialist and liaison psychiatrist who work with infants, children and adolescents. The stages of normal childhood development will be related to the particular needs of each age group in relation to hospitalization and surgery. Means for preventing undesirable psychological consequences in each age group will then be discussed.

For many years surgeons dealt with children and adolescents as if they were small adults. However, in the late 1930's and early 1940's, a large number of studies on child development began to affect general surgical care. Initially such studies emphasized the general emotional needs of childhood as the child moved from infancy through adolescence [4, 14, 18, 53, 56]. These studies were paralleled by research into the cognitive development of children [7, 24, 47].

Subsequent to these pioneering studies of child development, a number of investigators began to study the effects of hospitalization and surgery on young children [3, 52, 55]. They found that extended hospitalizations could cause severe depression and even death. As early as 1952 *Anna Freud* [18] speculated on the long-term effects of physical illness in children on psychological equilibrium in later life. As a result of these studies, increasing atten-

Table I. Stages of childhood development

Infancy:	0–15 months	prelocomotor	trust vs. mistrust
Toddler:	15–30 months	locomotor period, acquisition of words	autonomy vs. shame and doubt
Pre-school:	3– 6 years	language	initiative vs. guilt
Latency:	6–12 years	cognitive development	industry vs. inferiority
Adolescence:			
Early:	13–16 years	defining identity	individual independence
Mid:	16–18 years	at multiple levels	sexual independence
Late:	18–22 years	evolution of complex and abstract thinking	role definition

tion has been turned toward these issues and has profoundly influenced attitudes regarding even 'routine' procedures such as hernias and tonsillectomies. Indeed, due mainly to the increased understanding of children's needs, surgical interventions for such conditions as hernias, which at one time required a week's hospitalization, now require a 'hospitalization' of only twelve hours or less [5, 6, 20, 25, 32, 33, 37, 43].

As this new information was disseminated, further studies in hospitals were undertaken by other investigators [1, 2, 34, 42, 50, 51] on the short-term effects of stressful situations presented by surgery and hospitalization on the emotional and cognitive development of the child [10]. The overwhelming technical advances in medicine continued to stimulate interest on the impact of illness and surgery on the emerging personality.

Our understanding of normal and abnormal child development has continued to increase as well. More elaborate and careful research of such issues as temperament and coping styles has evolved, contributing to what we now know about children and their needs [16, 21, 27, 49].

The physician who deals directly with small children requires an understanding of the characteristics differentiating childhood from later periods. He/she needs to recognize the child's need for 'significant others' who ensure survival in light of limited ability to cope with external stresses without succumbing to disintegrative panic [15]. In addition, the doctor must understand that the child has an active fantasy life and a great deal of anxiety which the hospitalization exacerbates [11–13]. Perhaps of greatest significance to the surgeon is the concept of body image which evolves within the psychology of the individual throughout childhood and adolescence. Distortion and disruption of the body image concept can lead to serious difficulties and adjustment problems later in life [18, 19, 28, 54, 58]. Body image issues should therefore be dealt with in a fashion that minimizes harm as much as possible.

Finally, the major distinction between childhood and adolescence, on the one hand and adulthood on the other, is that during the first twenty or so years of life the individual is going through rapidly evolving developmental stages during which specific psychological tasks must be surmounted. For convenience, these periods of life are divided in the discussion below according to the psychological tasks that are most important for the child to complete. These essential stages of development and their approximate ages, according to *Erikson and Piaget*, are summarized in table I [14, 17]:

Infancy (0–15 months)

Infancy is a period during which the organism is totally dependent on its environment for surival. In this period, specific forms of attachment, stimulation and interaction with primary caretakers appear to be essential for normal development of trust and the prevention of retardation [4, 53, 56]. Investigators of the hospital scene in the 1940's and 1950's saw children in the hands of unfamiliar caretakers in traumatic circumstances, separated by long periods from 'significant others'. Their long-term studies indicated a powerful negative effect of antiquated visiting rules, extended hospitalizations and the resulting lack of physical stimulation [50, 52, 57]. Their findings have led to the current practices of sleeping-in by parents, shorter hospitalizations, early mobilizations and infant stimulation programs at most high quality medical and surgical centers. While some readers may view these practical efforts as established procedures today, there are still many hospitals that arbitrarily limit involvement of parents and have little in the way of infant stimulation programs. For many years medical and nusing staffs overtly struggled against liberalizing visiting hours because they considered the presence of visitors disruptive and inconvenient. Furthermore, infants who are separated from their parents appeared easier to handle, thus reinforcing staff attitudes. It was later discovered that these infants had become somewhat depressed, therefore quiet and withdrawn. Long-term separations can lead to 'hospitalism', mirasmus and death, phenomena that rarely occur in modern advanced settings [52, 56].

Except for the desirability of minimizing separation and strange environments, there is little else that is known about the appropriate psychological preparation for surgery in pre-verbal childern. In long-term follow-up, infants who have had adequate stimulation and association with their parents have shown none of the gross signs of deprivation reported in early studies. This does not mean that a major surgical experience early in life has no effect on personality development, but only that we have no clear notion of what the effect is. It may be that the brain of the immature infant provides a kind of protection to the developing organism that the child may lack in the following two periods of life [8, 21].

Toddler Stage (15–30 months)

The toddler stage is motorically very active. During this period, children are gaining control and use of all major voluntary motor systems. The psychological task associated with this period is that of defining autonomy versus shame and doubt. Speech is primitive and concrete with concepts simple [14, 17, 24]. Bad-good is of major concern to the toddler, and the primitive conscience forms during this period. In the toddler's world, therefore, confusing or painful medical procedures often become punishments for bad deeds. In addition, toddlers handle immobilization very poorly, becoming depressed very quickly [52]. Most of the early studies of immobilization due to hospitalization were gathered by investigators in rheumatic fever institutions for long-term care as well as orphanages and burn services where children were severely immobilized for long periods. While this kind of hospitalization is not completely analogous to the surgical circumstances, studies tend to make clear that early mobilization was salutory [23, 28, 36, 37, 41, 55]. Physical benefits of early mobilization post surgery (such as the prevention of emboli) were not discovered until many years after. Other investigators such as *Prugh* showed that convalescence was hastened by mobilization [49]. Since it was established early that toys play a particularly important role in the symbolic life of children at this stage of development, the 'transitional object', such as a favorite toy from home, was found to be an added benefit in the hospital setting [14, 52].

In this age group the child's verbal skills still remain inadequate to the task of dealing with trauma, pain, and the complexity of the medical environment. Usually any effort to communicate the need for staying still or follow-ing a preparation protocol for anesthesia results in panic and physical negativism. While the two-year-old is not capable of rational cooperation, he/she is, unfortunately, acutely enough aware of his/her surroundings to develop phobic behaviors which may last for significant periods post surgery. This 'white-coat syndrome' or fear of M.D.'s can last a lifetime. Children have great difficulty integrating traumatic experiences below the ages of seven to eight when the cognitive coping mechanisms of rationalization and intellectualization become usable and useful. This has led some authorities to strongly urge postponing surgery in childhood to the latest age possible. Certainly these recommendations had some influence in the 1950's when minor surgery for tonsils and adenoids were 'routine' in pre-school children [22, 31, 40, 46].

Pre-School Age (3–6 years)

Erikson [14] has called the next developmental stage the stage of initi-ative. Biological development, especially in the cognitive and language areas, progresses by leaps and bounds. Fine motor coordination increases to the point that drawing and writing letters become possible. In a sense, the end product is a being that can communicate and begin to function indepen-dently in the outside world with guidance from any adult, rather than a pri-mary parent or surrogate. The child has available new coping styles; commu-nication can become meaningful, not just 'baby talk'.

Curiosity to understand the world and the self become exceedingly important to the child as does the human body, the body image, and human sexuality. Indeed, concerns and conflicts around bodily integrity, separation, and independence characterize the oedipal period. Such concerns arise out of the cognitive ability to understand concepts around how the body works, why there are differences in people, and how one finds out about these issues. The period begins with an organism that has many unformed, unrealistic, and magical fantasies [18]. Hopefully it ends with a child who is beginning to be independent and has a reasonable grasp of reality [14, 17].

Because so much of this period seems to involve the cognitive task of differentiating fantasy from reality, physicians must be prepared to commu-nicate more directly and openly with patients over age three. Most profes-sionals believe that while language and cognition may still be limited in the pre-school child, his/her fantasies are always worse than any reality that has to be consciously dealt with. Thus while it is not necessary to describe to the child what will happen while asleep on the operating table, it now becomes increasingly important to detail exactly what will happen in the hospital before and after surgery. Most early studies indicated that parents, relatives and physicians have erred in the direction of either communicating too little to patients at all age levels or else of communicating in technical 'jargonese'.

The best tertiary-care settings now have pre-surgical preparation programs [48]. They are available to all children in every age group whose parents are willing to have their children attend. The better programs are usually run by nurses and child life personnel and include slide lectures or puppet shows as well as tours of the hospital facilities (including recovery room and ICU's when the child is expected to be *conscious* in such a setting). Often the children are allowed to actually play with real equipment if it will be used on them, e.g., masks, oxygen tents, stethoscopes, blood pressure cuffs, and encouraged to ask any and all questions that come to mind. Quite frightening distortions and expectations, such as smothering in an oxygen tent, can be dealt with [9, 22]. While the programs described above tend to exist primarily at large, tertiary-care children's hospitals, many smaller hospitals have introduced coloring books, show-and-tell books, or other simple reality-testing aids as part of the admission process.

These younger age groups still have difficulty integrating the total experience of surgery according to some data. However both short-term and long-term studies appear to confirm that children are better able to deal with these experiences if they are realistically prepared for the experience and are able to play out any distortions as well as ventilate questions, fantasies and feelings afterwards [25, 44, 45, 59]. (P. 23 deals further with outcomes of psychological interventions in pre-surgical patients.)

Because pre-school children are still too young to do without 'significant others' (parents, etc.) for very long, one member or another of the family is encouraged to remain even at night for most or all of the hospitalization. This practice relates to psychoanalytic theories of unconscious and conscious oedipal guilt thought to be generated in children from the age of three on. Thus, some children are felt to have problems integrating illness and surgery without feeling that they are being punished for some prior 'badness' or 'evil thought'. Some theorists feel this is a greater problem with children getting surgery for 'asymptomatic' conditions. It is believed that having a reassuring parent around much of the time tends to mitigate some of this guilty feeling, especially in the younger child who usually has great difficulty in understanding that physical pathology can exist without any personal control or involvement in its existence. Such feelings often exist in adults as well (was it something I ate, drank, or did?) and are good examples of the persistence of what is called magical thinking [18].

Latency (6–12 years)

Between the ages of about six through twelve there is a relatively easy-to-manage period which psychoanalysts call the latency age. *Erikson* [14] indicated that children at this age are concerned with industry, as opposed to inferiority. Developmentally this is a period of great intellectual and social growth. It is a period when children determine their emotional, social, intellectual and physical strengths and weaknesses. They begin to identify with a wide variety of 'culture heroes', whose characteristics become blended into the child's individual personality. Children's hunger for information and our society's tendency to view health professionals as 'culture heroes' can contribute to both smoother preparation for, and management through, a surgical experience. Also since children now have greater independence, parents can usually spend some time away from the hospital after the first, more critical days post-operation. This usually translates to 24 hours after returning to a ward on full convalescent status.

All children in this age group should clearly be involved in preparation for hospitalization and direct, simple explanations of their problems and the why and hows of 'fixing' them. They also ought to be able to practice for post-surgical recovery room and ICU tasks such as balloon blowing, respiratory exercises, and coughing. Children of this age take poorly to careless communications ('this won't hurt a bit', etc.). Often physicians will unnecessarily turn a child who wishes to be cooperative into an angry resister. Latency age children want to be liked, therefore will make efforts to please the adults around them [14, 26].

Most studies appear to indicate that children from 8 to 12 have fewer coping problems in the hospital and fewer long-term psychological problems post-surgery than any age group up to late adolescence. This resilience probably has a number of complicated causes. First, reality testing after age eight is quite sophisticated and body image is now integrated into the personality. Furthermore, educational experience including television has made children more sophisticated than ever before about doctors, hospitals and medicine. In addition, any intervention that improves physical function dovetails directly into the developmental needs in this period, as our culture tends to reward any improved physical or 'sports' function. Obviously, to be able to play better and longer, to look more 'normal', to be more coordinated all reinforce the goals of being good at something and striving for improvement. Thus almost any type of cardiac, plastic, orthopedic, or neurosurgery tends to have some positive aspects to compensate for the pain, trauma, and scarring that can result [21, 27, 35].

Certain aspects of preparation and care that are normally most appropriate to the younger age groups may sometimes have to be considered for a latency or older child because of immaturity or special needs (retardation, prior emotional problems) [7]. Under some circumstances children in this age group can occasionally benefit from early surgery, rather than waiting until adolescence with its more complicated physical and developmental tasks [9].

Adolescence (13–22 years)

As latency moves into puberty and puberty into adolescence, there are a host of new psychological concerns and developmental tasks. *Erikson* conceptualizes adolescence as a period during which identity is formed; *Piaget* considers it a period in which abstract thought and concepts develop; others have written about it as a time of turmoil and conflict [14, 17]. Most psychological change is believed to be accompanied by profound biochemical and biological changes involved with puberty. These changes are particularly pronounced with the establishment of secondary sexual characteristics and the maturation of procreational functions. The psychology of the adolescent has complicated implications for surgical preparation and management, as will be discussed below.

Adolescence stretches chronologically from about age 13 to the early twenties when the individual becomes self-supporting or at least completely independent from parents. Depending on the culture, this period can be shortened or extended depending on the circumstances. In American society, adolescence covers approximately age 13 to 22 (the end of college). The adolescent's struggle for identity divides itself relevantly into three periods that overlap but highlight problems of significance to the surgeon.

Since the adolescent is especially involved in identity formation and can now think more abstractly, as a general rule it is important to begin to discuss a broader set of issues with him/her. Furthermore, because issues of informed consent (depending on the state) arise after the age of fourteen, broader discussion with the patient is very important in gaining trust and cooperation. In addition, for developmental reasons (see next section) it becomes increasingly important to spend some time with the patient alone, according him/her some respect as an individual. The closer the patient is to a majority age, the more important this is, especially if one wants an accurate history. Adolescents have secrets and personal lives. They will almost never reveal a drug or sexual history with parents present. In some surgical situations data of this kind may be extraordinarily important [30].

Early Adolescence (13–16 years)

The initial psychological issue that is relevant to identity formation is the adolescent's need to become individually free (independent) from his/her parents. Thus the period from age 13 to 16 is often somewhat strife-torn especially around issues such as staying out at night, when and how to do homework. Clearly, above the age of 14 the patient should be nominally made part of the decision-making process. Then if the adolescent agrees to the surgery with parents present, a discussion of preparation for surgery can ensue. Individual one-to-one discussion should take place. More than the usual time should be spent allowing an adolescent to ask questions and get details about pain, mobilization, freedom of motion, and activity. The more immature the adolescent, the more likely that techniques for the 'under twelve' child may be useful. However, even the mature adolescent will have great difficulty with dependency and 'rule following' at this time. Major surgery is best done at institutions equiped with activity areas designed for adolescents and staffed by physicians and nurses willing to accept some struggles for independence in this age group. The surgeon who works with adolescents must remain flexible and patient, explaining his/her reasons for enforced immobilization or 'special rules' following surgery to the adolescent [30, 41, 48].

Other aspects of independent indentity that become important during early adolescence are new conflicts around body image. Obviously, surgery, even of a minor nature, is scarrifying; a two-inch appendectomy scar can loom as large as the San Andreas fault in the mind's eye of a 15 year old. 'How will it look afterwards?' should always be discussed, even if the patient is too intimidated or anxious to ask. Often, professionals forget how bad even 'beautiful plastic surgery scars' look the first few days after the operation, and how well they look in the long run. Some studies have indicated that large scars in adolescents can take a very long time to heal psychologically. Last, but not at all least, is the need to respect the rapid development of modesty during this period. The need for modesty represents a significant problem in large teaching hospitals and must be dealt with on an individual basis. A clear policy of adequate 'draping' during examinations usually precludes potential embarrassment and should not be forgotten. Attention to such details often avoids angry confrontations and lack of cooperation on the part of adolescent patients [8, 21, 30].

For the young adolescent, relationships with parents are often quite ambivalent and occasionally stormy. While it is still reasonable to have parents around 24 hours a day in the ICU and recovery room, parents need not be present as often during convalescence. The adolescents themselves are often the best people to communicate their needs; the physician often has to help the patient get the parents to accommodate (i.e., get out). Often parents will infantilize in a guilty way and will need encouragement to leave [30].

Mid-Adolescent (15–18 years)

For the patient in the middle adolescent period (15–18 years), sexual identity is a complex issue that becomes incorporated in the development. Concomitant with this developing sexuality and partly because of it, the adolescent has an increased investment in peer-group ideals, standards and functions. At the same time that the adolescent is working through individual problems of independence and sexual identity, he/she is highly sensitive to group values: special interests, special dances (such as rock 'n' roll), eating fads, clothing and speech that are particular to each generation.

By this age, pre-surgical and post-surgical discussions should primarily involve a one-to-one relationship between surgeon and patients, with the parents a somewhat secondary consideration. Usually, this orientation is not respected and often leads to disagreements and lack of cooperation, it can lead to outright refusal of surgery [30].

Given the concerns of this age group, it is important to address diplomatically issues around sexuality while preparing a patient for surgery. Despite modern sexual enlightment and activity, numerous studies have confirmed that adolescents are very ignorant about sexual anatomy and physiology. Thus any abdominal or genito-urinary surgery will cause fears and conflicts. Indeed surgery may be resisted unless the adolescent is reassured that the operation will not cause sterility, impotence, frigidity, etc. If it will, considerable counseling may be in order.

Surgical procedures that will result in long-term impairment of physical function and educational loss should be addressed as early as possible [2, 26]. While such discussion is always necessary, it is especially so for this age group. The inability to function on an equal footing with one's peers always leads to loss of self-esteem. Such feelings often lead to depression and potentially even more serious sequellae [11]. (Suicide is now the number three killer of adolescents between 16 and 25 – no surgical mortality comes close to it.)

While the surgeon does not personally need to manage loss of function pre- and post-surgery, it is his/her responsibility to mobilize all the rehabilitative forces necessary to deal with the problem as soon as surgically permissible. Most tertiary-care settings are set up to deal with such problems, since most of the major elective impairing surgery in this age group is oncological in nature (amputations for sarcomas and neurosurgical tumor surgery). Studies in the field of general hospital psychiatry indicate overwhelmingly that even young patients should be informed of impairing surgery and have a chance to talk about it to professional personnel for a day or two beforehand if possible [29]. Many tertiary-care hospitals have specially trained nurses, social workers or liaison psychiatrists available for counseling after the surgeon talks to the patient about the impending loss of limb or function. The antiquated approach which allowed patients to 'find out for themselves' post-operatively no longer appears to be psychologically, morally, or even legally viable for almost any age [11, 30].

In preparing an adolescent for amputation, the surgical staff must plan to initiate early mobilization. Such preparation allows the patient to approach a level of function consistent with that of his/her peers faster than the unprepared patient, may prevent or moderate any concomitant loss of self-esteem, and can minimize the potential for catastrophic and sometimes fatal post-operative reactions [35]. (Limb amputation is discussed further on p. 200.)

Undoubtedly adolescents in this period handle benign surgery worse than any other age group except the three- to six-year olds. Probably the adolescent's stresses in the social, sexual, and intellectual arenas, the push to college, and getting away from one's parents leave little room for the additional stress of surgery. Resistance and negativism should not be considered abnormal in this age group. Calm and considerate counseling, plus possibly postponing the operation, will often be enough to get the patient to accept and cooperate in a surgical effort [30].

There is one small caution to be mentioned during this period and perhaps the next. Facial and breast surgery should be thoroughly discussed with patient and family, especially in situations where the surgeon sees little to confirm the adolescent's self dislike. Mid-adolescence especially is a time of ambivalence and distortion of fantasy life; surgery can occasionally appear to be a solution to social and peer-group relationship problems. Such distortions always lead to difficulties after the operation, when it is too late to change directions [30, 35]. (Cosmetic surgery is further discussed on p. 84.)

Late Adolescence (18–22 years)

The oldest adolescents are obviously in their legal majority and must be dealt with directly. Clearly, informed consent is a necessity, as is a thorough discussion of the long-term implications of surgery. In a sense, the major identity issue of this period is that of 'role' identity – which, therefore, includes some of the issues of the period before and integrates them into those of career and parenting. Thus, surgery may have major impact on the individual's long-term goals and plans and may lead to serious psychological difficulty.

Psychological preparation and immediate post-operative management may be similar to that of the typical adult. (This is discussed further on p. 23.) Major career issues must be addressed. While the surgeon may most appropriately coordinate efforts of other staff rather than directly attempting counseling, major career concerns are almost universal in adolescents undergoing surgery for trauma, cancer, sports injury (for serious athletes) or problems involving sexual organs. Again, rehabilitative efforts should be initiated rapidly, effectively, and comprehensively. Those institutions without such resources probably should avoid major surgical efforts.

Conclusion

A few words should be addressed to two areas in which there is a relative lack of knowledge concerning long-term sequelae and stresses, that is, severe burn and transplant surgery in children and adolescents. Since the long-term management of these patients has not been primarily surgical and there are few if any groups large enough to generalize about, current principles of dealing with recurrent surgery and chronic disease tend to be utilized [9, 30, 50].

As a final caution, psychiatric epidemiologists point out that from the age of fifteen upwards, mental illness related to biological vulnerability, such as the severe breakdowns seen in schizophrenia and bipolar disease, begin a rapidly rising curve that peaks in young adulthood. While psychotic breaks in a hospitalized patient cannot be predicted with accuracy, it is becoming more and more important that surgeons take careful detailed histories of psychological development in order to prevent such occurrences [39]. If a patient has a prior history of serious psychological disability, appropriate mental health professionals can be involved to work closely with the adolescent, thereby minimizing potential difficulties and stresses [29].

References

1   Blanton, S.; Kirk, R.: A psychiatric study of sixty-one appendectomy cases. Ann. Surg. *126:* 305 (1947).

2   Blotchky, M.J.; Grossman, I.: Psychological implications of childhood genitourinary surgery. J. Am. Acad. Child Psychiat. *31:* 488 (1978).

3   Bowlby, J.; Robertson, J.; Rosenbluth, D.: A two year old goes to the hospital. Psychoanalyt. Study Child *7:* 82 (1952).

4   Bowlby, J.: Attachment and Loss. Vol. 1 (Hogarth Press, London 1969).

5   Bothe, A.; Galdston, R.: The child's loss of consciousness: A psychiatric view of pediatric anesthesia. Pediatrics *60:* 252 (1972).

6   Cenmak, E.G.; Brutt, M.M.: Behavior changes indicating emotional trauma in tonsillectomized children. Pediatrics *12:* 23 (1953).

7   Cline, F.W.; Rothenberg, M.B.: Preparation of a child for major surgery: A case report. J. Am. Acad. Child Psychiat. *13:* 78 (1978).

8   Danilowicz, D.A.; Gabriel, H.P.: Postoperative reactions in children: 'normal' and abnormal reaction after cardiac surgery. Am. J. Psychiat. *128:* 185 (1971).

9   Danilowicz, D.A.; Gabriel, H.P.: Responses of children to cardiac surgery. Psychiatric Aspects of Surgery, Howells. Vol. 7, pp. 267–284 (Brunner/Mazel, New York 1976).

10   Davenport, H.T.: Werry, J.S.: The effect of general anesthesia, surgery, and hospitalization upon the behavior of children. Am. J. Orthopsychiat. *40:* 806 (1970).

11   Drotar, D.: The treatment of a severe anxiety reaction in an adolescent boy following renal transplantation. J. Am. Acad. Child Psychiat. *14:* 451 (1975).

12   Egerton, N.; Kay, J.H.: Psychological disturbances associated with open heart surgery. Br. J. Psychiat. *110:* 443 (1964).

13   Eickenhoff, J.E.; Kneale, D.H.; Dripps, R.D.: Incidence and etiology of postanesthetic excitement. Anesthesiology *22:* 667 (1961).

14   Erikson, E.: Childhood and Society. (W.W. Norton and Co., Inc., New York 1963).

15   Fagin, C.M.: The effects of maternal attendance during hospitalization on the post-hospital behavior of young children: A comparative study (Davis, Philadelphia 1966).

16   Falstein, E.I.; Judas, I.; Mendelsolin, R.: Fantasies in children prior to herniorraphy. Am. J. Orthopsychiat. *27:* 800 (1957).

17   Flavel, J.N.: The developmental psychology of Jean Piaget (Van Nostrand, Princeton 1963).

18   Fraiberg, S.H.: The Magic Years (Scribner's, New York 1959).
19   Freud, A.: The role of bodily illness in the mental life of children. Psychoanalyt. Study
      Child 7: 69–81 (1952).
20   Gabriel, H.P.: A practical approach to preparing children for dermatol. Surg. Oncol. 3:
      523–526 (1977).
21   Gabriel, H.P.; Danilowicz, D.: Post-operative responses in the 'prepared' child after car-
      diac surgery. Brit. Heart J. 40: 1046 (1978).
22   Gabriel, H.P.; Danilowicz, D.A.: Open Heart Surgery for Congenital Heart Disease:
      Minimizing Adverse Psychological Sequelae in Families Facing Major High-risk Surgery.
      Psychosocial Family Interventions in Pediatric Illness, pp. 103–114 (Plenum Publishing
      Co., New York 1982).
23   Gladston, R.: The burning and the healing of children; in Chess and Thomas, Annual
      progress child psychiatry and child development (Brunner/Mazel, New York 1974).
24   Gesel, A.: The first five years of life: A guide to the study of the preschool child (Harper
      and Bros, New York 1940).
25   Goldman, H.; Bohcali, A.: Psychological preparation of children for tonsillectomy. Laryn-
      goscope 76: 1698 (1966).
26   Gross, R.E.; Jewett, T.C., Jr.: Surgical experiences from 1,222 operations for undescended
      testes. J. Am. med. Ass. 160: 634 (1956).
27   Hamburg, D.; Hamburg, B.; De Goz, S.: Adaptive problems and mechanisms in the se-
      verely burned patient. Psychiatry 16: 1 (1953).
28   Healy, M.H.; Hansen, H.: Psychiatric management of the limb amputation in a preschool
      child: The illusion of like me – not me. J. Am. Acad. Child Psychiat. 16: 684 (1977).
29   Hockaday, W.J.: Experiences of a psychiatrist as a member of a surgical faculty. Am. J.
      Psychiat. 117: 706 (1961).
30   Hofman, A.D.; Becker, R.D.; Gabriel, H.P.: The Hospitalized Adolescent: A Guide for
      Managing the Ill and Injured Youth (Free Press, Riverside, 1976).
31   Jackson, K.: Psychologic preparation as a method of reducing the emotional trauma of
      anesthesia in children Anesthesiology 12: 293 (1951).
32   James, F.E.: The behavior reactions of normal children to common operations. Practi-
      tioner 185: 339 (1960).
33   Jessner, L.; Blos, G.E.; Waldfogel, S.: Emotional implications of tonsillectomy and
      adenoidectomy on children. Psychoanalyt. Study Child 7: 126 (1952).
34   Jongkees, L.B.W.: The psychic effect of hospital and surgical interventions on children.
      Am. Ontol. Rhinol. Larynogol. 63: 145 (1954).
35   Jorring, K.: Amputation in children. Acta Orthopsychiat. Scand. 42: 178 (1971).
36   Korsch, B.M.; et al.: Experience with children and their families during extended
      hemodialysis and kidney transplantation. Pediat. Clin. North Am. 18: 625 (1971).
37   Korsch, B.M.; et al.: Kidney transplantation in children: Psychosocial follow-up study. J.
      Pediatr. 88: 399 (1973).
38   Lawrie, R.: Operating on children as day cases. Lancet 2: 1289 (1964).
39   Lazarus, H.R.; Hagens, J.H.: Prevention of psychosis following open-heart surgery. Am.
      J. Psychiat. 124: 1190 (1968).
40   Levy, D.M.: Psychic trauma of operations in children and a note on combat neurosis. Am.
      J. Dis. Child 69: 7 (1945).
41   Loomis, E.: The child's emotions and surgery; in Kiesewetter, Pre- and post-operative care
      in the pediatric surgical patient (Year Book, Chicago 1956).

42   Mattsson, A.: Long-term physical illness in childhood: A challenge to psychosocial adaptation. Pediatrics, *50:* 801–811 (1972).

43   McKee, W.J.E.: Controlled study of the effects of tonsillectomy and adenoidectomy in children. Brit. J. Prev. Soc. Med. *17:* 49 (1963).

44   McKeith, R.: Children in hospital: Preparation for operation. Lancet *2:* 843 (1953).

45   Melish, R.W.P.: Preparation of a child for hospitalization and surgery. Pediatr. Clin. North Am. *16:* 543 (1969).

46   Pearson, G.H.J.: Effect of operative procedures on the emotional life of the child. Am. J. Dis. Child *62:* 716 (1941).

47   Piaget, J.: The Origins of Intelligence in Children (International Universities Press, New York, 1952).

48   Potts, W.J.: The surgeon and the child (Saunders, Philadelphia 1956).

49   Prugh, D.G.; Staub, E.; Sands, H.H.; Kirschbaum, R.M.; Lenihan, E.A.: A study of the emotional reactions of children and families to hospitalization and illness. Am. J. Orthopsychiat. *23:* 70–106 (1953).

50   Prugh, D.G.: Emotional reactions to surgery; in the non-operative aspects of surgery. Report of the Twenty-Seventh Ross Conference on Pediatric Research (Ross Labs, Columbus 1958).

51   Prugh, D.G.; Eckhardt, L.O.: Preparing children psychologically for painful medical and surgical procedures; in Gilbert, Psychosocial aspects of pediatric care (Grune and Stratton, New York 1978).

52   Robertson, J.: Young children in hospital (Basic Books, New York 1958, 1970).

53   Rutter, M.: Maternal Deprivation Revisited (Penguin Books, Harmondsworth, England 1974).

54   Siller, J.: Psychological concomitants of amputation in children. Child Dev. *31:* 109 (1960).

55   Spitz, R.A.: Hospitalism: An inquiry into the genesis of psychiatric conditions in early childhood. Psychoanalyt. Study Child *1:* 153–174 (1946).

56   Spitz, R.A.; Wolf, K.M.: Anaclitic depression: An inquiry into the genesis of psychiatric conditions in early childhood. Psychoanalytic Study of the Child *2:* 313 (1946).

57   Toker, E.: Psychiatric aspects of cardiac surgery in a child. J. Am. Acad. Child Psychiat. *10:* 156 (1981).

58   Tourkow, L.: Psychic consequences of loss and replacement of body parts. J. Am. Psychoanalyt. Assoc. *22:* 170 (1974).

59   Visintainer, M.A.; Wolfer, J.A.: Psychological preparation for surgical pediatric patients: The effect on children's and parents' stress responses and adjustment. Pediatrics *56:* 187 (1975).

H. Paul Gabriel, MD, Department of Psychiatry, New York University Medical Center, New York, NY 10016 (USA)

Adv. psychosom. Med., vol. 15, pp. 84–108 (Karger, Basel 1986)

Psychological Effects of Aesthetic Facial Surgery

Marcia Kraft Goin, John M. Goin

University of Southern California School of Medicine, Los Angeles, Calif., USA

To understand the scope of this chapter, some definitions need to be kept in mind. Plastic surgery is a broad surgical speciality that is unique in that it is not limited to an organ system or systems, as are urology, neurosurgery, orthopedic surgery and cardiovascular surgery. It is a speciality concerned with the surgery of repair, largely (but by no means entirely) of the surface of the body. Plastic surgeons operate on bones, tendons, nerves, muscle and blood vessels as well as skin. Their area of competence extends from the scalp to the soles of the feet. The field includes the surgery of cancer, trauma, burns, chronic wounds, congenital anomalies and appearance. This last area, aesthetic (or cosmetic) surgery is often confused with the speciality as a whole.

Aesthetic surgery has been defined as 'surgery which is designed to correct defects which the average prudent observer would consider to be within the range of normal'. Successful aesthetic surgery, then, must improve upon the normal. The expectation is that this goal will be reached. In contrast, reconstructive surgery is designed to bring the abnormal closer to normality. A complete restoration of the normal is rarely achieved, regardless of the magnitude of the 'defect'; a small scar, a cleft lip, or a lower jaw removed for cancer. But aesthetic surgery regularly improves on the normal. The following two cases illuminate issues relevant to a psychiatrist's understanding of aesthetic surgery.

Mrs. K. has had a face-lift. She has healed well. Her appearance is improved but not strikingly so; she was not a terribly good candidate for the operation in the first place. Her older sister maintains that she sees little change. Her 25-year-old daughter tells her that she looks marvelous. She has changed her hair style and is dressing more fashionably. She has been asked to serve on the Board of the Community Cancer Center and the seemingly diminishing prospects of promotion to Vice-President of the bank where she works now seem brighter. She says that the face-lift is the best thing that she has ever done. In gratitude, she gives her surgeon a tiny and incredibly complicated LED travel alarm clock that he can't seem to operate.

Mr. B. has had a rhinoplasty. He has healed well. His before and after photographs show a dramatic improvement. His surgeon is pleased. The surgeon's staff compliments him on his technical achievement. Mr. B. however, is desperately unhappy. He says that his nose seems to belong to someone else. It looks 'plastic'. People stare at him in the street. They suppress smiles at the obviousness of his 'nose job'. Certain angles are wrong. It is difficult to explain. He thinks of nothing else. He visits his surgeon weekly. Each time his name appears on the day sheet, the surgeon's stomach sinks. 'You've got to do something', Mr. B. says. 'There is nothing to do', the surgeon says, 'your nose looks great. Give it a rest for a few months, you'll get used to it.' One night Mr. B. appears in the emergency department. He is obviously 'on' something or another. His speech is slurred but he is able to ask that his surgeon be called. With a razor blade he has sliced off part of the tip of his nose. The cartilages are exposed. A skin graft may be required. Mr. B. has successfully recaptured his surgeon's attention.

Why should this be? How can two straightforward aesthetic operations performed by a technically skilled surgeon end up so differently? Although all the answers are not in; there is a large body of data (some hard, some soft) that give us a reasonably sound basis for understanding these extraordinarily different responses to desired and well-wrought changes in the body. Parenthetically, these two brief case reports were not concocted; they are real, and similar reactions occur with sufficient frequency in the practice of plastic surgery to make most plastic surgeons greatly concerned about the proper selection of patients and deeply aware of the unexploded psychological bombs that may lie beneath apparently placid surfaces.

Those who are relatively unconcerned about their appearance often find it difficult to understand someone's decision to have a face-lift, a rhinoplasty, or some other operation which is intended to change and improve appearance. Many believe that the desire to change a surface appearance reflects a superficiality in that person's personality, a vanity, an emptiness, a self-centered narcissism. They have never thought much about the intimate connection between one's sense of self and one's feelings about one's body. Instead, it is assumed that cultural influences, fashion and 'the media' create an emphasis on 'the beautiful people' and that these and other purely social factors lead people to elect to have such operations.

Yet, psychiatrists have long been aware of the fact that operations that change a body part can have a potent effect on the psyche. Early papers on the subject [1, 2] described patients who developed psychological disturbances after such changes. Later studies have shown that the reverse could also be true. While patients desiring a rhinoplasty seem to be more disturbed than the general population, on the average certain of their MMPI scores actually improve following surgery. [3]

Body and Body Image – Developmental Issues

Feelings, conscious and unconscious, about the body are a powerful psychological force. As a consequence, one person adjusting to a sudden change in a body part may develop serious psychological problems while another may show a dramatically positive psychological response. Body image, the psychological picture of the body in one's mind's eye, is a strong and essential part of the experience of an integrated sense of self. Consequently, changes which affect the body image have similar psychological potency. (Body image is further discussed on p. 200, Sequelae of limb amputation.)

As *Freud* [4] said, 'the ego is first and foremost a bodily ego; it is not merely a surface, but is itself a projection of the surface'. Newborns come into the world with certain constitutional and genetically determined physical attributes, but their psychic structures are amorphous. They experience the world through sensations. The cruelty of the world equates with hunger pangs while the warmth a simple satisfaction of nursing is experienced as a world of comfort. A newborn does not experience the nurturing warmth that is its mother as a separate being but rather as part of the self; the two are at first inseparably merged and without boundaries. As the baby matures, and begins to reach out and touch and see, an awareness dawns that the self and the nurturing entity are actually separate. This early consciousness of separatness evokes anxiety, a sense of danger and vulnerability linked with the possibility of being abandoned. In this 'six months anxiety' we can see the first evidences of the psychological effects of one aspect of the body image: awareness of body boundaries, and the anxiety attendant with the beginning of the phase of separation and individuation. [5]

Mahler's [6] report on the responses of infants to their reflected images seems relevant to our understanding of the significance of one's mirrored reflection. Her data show that infants first explore themselves and others with their hands. Then, beginning around six months they become interested in and excited by their mirrored reflections. By eight months of age they appear to be less interested in touching their own body parts and more excited by looking at themselves in the mirror. The authors considered it noteworthy that the excitement elicited by mirroring feedback was 'especially marked in, more important to, and also more actively sought by, babies in whom the mother's investment had been poor' [6, p. 840]. *Kohut* has underscored the need for infants to see love and acceptance mirrored in the faces of their mothers. He theorizes that infants deprived of this mirrored approval grow up with severe emotional deficits. During treatment attempts to create this sense of acceptance simulate the development of the 'mirror transference' [7].

Mahler's data support this theory and explain the importance of one's reflection in normal development. It may also explain the hypertrophied importance of appearance for those with poor early nurturing. In other words, those infants with inadequate mothering grow up with an intense longing for acceptance and approval from those who become important to them. Failing to find it there, they may have to search ceaselessly for it in their own mirrored reflections. As they grow older they look in the mirror for that sense of internal security which they have failed to find in others. The message of the mirror may provoke the emotional need for an aesthetic operation. The emotional significance of an operation may in turn become linked with internal security. Post-operatively the 'mirror, mirror on the wall' will be consulted to see if they are not only 'fairest of them all' but most secure as well.

This is not to assert or imply that all concerns about appearance are the result of early reactions to separation anxiety or responses to inadequate mothering. But the psychological importance of the body and its reflection originates at a very early stage of psychological development. The extent of this early influence will depend upon each individual's early experience. Thereafter, innumerable other experiences will affect the self-perception of the body as one proceeds up the ladder of *Erickson's* psychosocial stages of development [8]. Beauty then, is in a sense often in the eye of the beheld, rather than in the eye of the beholder.

Reactions to the Face

The responses of others also play their part. In nursery school, pretty children are the most coveted playmates. Studies [9] have shown that teachers tend to judge misbehavior as 'just a phase' in attractive children and 'definite social problems' in homely ones. Familial experiences may be as important as intrapsychic and cultural factors.

Two contrasting rhinoplasty patients, described in our study [10], illustrate this. A young man told his psychiatrist: 'My nose looks like my father's. I hate him, I hate it, and I want it changed.' Following his rhinoplasty he was pleased with the new shape of his nose and became more self-confident. A young woman was happy with the physical result of the rhinoplasty but felt a deep sense of loss because she no longer resembled her beloved father. Surgical changes of facial features, particularly the nose, can result in feelings of separation from the family or in the loss of identification with a cultural or ethnic heritage. How the individual feels about the family or the ethnic group will affect the psychological impact of the operation and the concomitant loss.

The face has a special meaning, exposed as it is for all the world to see. *Meerloo* [11] has described the face as the 'label' of 'character' and ethnic background. The face also conveys, through expressions and animations real and perceived, the emotional state of the individual. Happiness, sadness, grief and anger are often difficult to hide. The emotion-portraying function of the face led a widow to request a face-lift so that she would 'look better' This was an expression of her hope that the operation would enable her to conceal the external manifestations of her grief. Another woman, angry and frightened by her husband's long and serious illness, wanted a face-lift to 'look refreshed'. What she really desired was to conceal her rage and frustration. As a mask to 'unacceptable' feelings, the operation made both of these women more comfortable and helped them to function more effectively in the undesired roles that life had thrust upon them.

In this brief overview of the many psychological forces which affect people's feelings about their bodies and body images, the complexity of psychological results begins to become apparent.

Patients Seeking Aesthetic Facial Surgery

It is impossible to make generalizations about the total population of aesthetic facial surgery patients. People of different age groups, sexes, ethnic groups, and psychological status tend to seek different operations and for different reasons. The painfully shy, introverted teenager with a large hooked nose who wants a rhinoplasty so that she can at last burst out of her psychic chrysalis has very little in common with the tough, leathery real-estate sales-woman who wants a face-lift because 'there are so many aggressive, good-looking younger women' in her field. Generalizations about people who request a particular operation, however, can be made and do have some validity.

Buhler [12, 13] described a number of characteristics that help people to cope with stresses of middle age. Among these were good self-esteem, having a variety of interests, a flexible attitude toward other people, a realistic view of one's personal capacities, and a willingness to accept help from others. Our own studies [14, 15] and those of *Webb* et al. [16] have shown face-lift patients to be notably deficient in many of these qualities.

Face-Lift Patients

Webb's et al. data were published in 1965, and reflect modes and social attitudes now nearly 20 years old. Their average face-lift patients was a 48 year old married, white protestant woman who was a reasonably affluent high-school graduate, and a product of what they called 'upper middle class'. Her personal life was stable. She had married before she was 29 and was still married to the same man. She was usually employed, though not the main source of financial support of her family. She had high aspirations, was activ-ity-minded, socially poised and tended to maintain somewhat superficial relations with others. In fact, there seemed to be two distinct patterns which these patients followed in their involvement with others. One group showed a tendency to form deeply dependent relations with a very few people, usu-ally a spouse or some other family member. The other group was distrustful of others and made only distant social contacts. They were self-centered, emotionally labile and failed to make deep emotional commitments to oth-ers.

Psychopathology was assessed in the 72 patients in this study group. 48 of these were referred for psychiatric consultation, and psychiatric diagnoses were made in 70% of them. Most of the psychiatric diagnosis were not of major pathology; rather they usually were: emotionally unstable personality, neurotic depressive reaction or passive dependent personality. 15 of the entire study group of 72 had undergone previous psychiatric treatment for mild to moderate emotional disturbances. One had a history of an acute paranoid schizophrenic reaction.

The younger patients in *Webb's* group seemed to have (and to have had in the past) more problems with personal adjustment and more significant family disruptions during childhood than the older patients. This finding led to an analysis of the psychological patterns of the patients and categorization into three age-related groups: the emotionally dependent group, the worker group, and the grief group. *Baker* [17, 18], a plastic surgeon who had reported on a series of 1500 face-lift patients, has commented that, '(this) grouping seems quite accurate and annoyingly consistent although at first glance it appears to be based on age.'

The emotionally dependent group comprised 21% of the sample, and were mainly between ages 29 and 39. They had repeated difficulties in meeting adult responsibilities and were very insecure. Those who were married were extremely dependent on their spouses while those who were widowed were 'shattered' by their losses and were unable to develop new relationships. Those with children found the parental role difficult to assume and tended to relate to their children childishly, as though they were siblings. Many felt simultaneously hostile and dependent toward their own parents.

Those in the worker group made up 37% of the sample, with most between the ages of 40 and 50. They were deeply committed to their careers. Their relationships were stable but rather distant. Their most significant relationships were often with co-workers. This group showed greater anxiety and ambivalence about aging than the other two.

As the name indicates, the grief group was characterized by the prevalence of grief reactions. They represented 42% of *Webb* et al.'s study sample (60% of our series [15] were in this age group). 90% of the patients in this group had lost an important person in their lives within the past 5 years. Definite signs of continuing grief were found in 60%. In contrast to the younger patients, those in the grief group were described as 'hyperindependent'. They regarded the acceptance of help from others as a sign of weakness. Hospital and office personnel often described these patients as 'cute and lively'. One of them articulated the grief group creed in this way: 'I want no sympathy. I want to succeed. I want to succeed so that I can turn around and help other people. I've played this role all my life. I don't want anything from anybody.'

When *Webb* et al. compared the psychological profiles of some randomly chosen face-lift patients with those of a control group, the face-lift patients were more likely to be suffering from grief, loneliness, depression and loss. They were also more fearful of intimacy and dependence, ambivalent about their parents and more concerned about aging and the possibility of abandonment. Personal achievement was more important to them than to the control group and they felt that their physical appearance did not mirror their true characters.

Two predominant personality patterns emerged from our own prospective study [15] of 50 female face-lift patients. One group tended to be aggressive, assertive, and energetic women who often showed poor judgement in social or sexual situations. Those in the second group appeared to be extroverted and socially outgoing but maintained a certain superficiality in their personal relationships. 66% had normal scores on the MMPI (Minnesota Multiphasic Personality Inventory). The others had mildly abnormal MMPIs showing such diagnostic tendencies such as impulsive character disorders, passive-aggressive personality, hysterical personality, etc. None was psychotic. About half had high expectations of themselves, were perfectionistic and were unable to admit to mistakes.

Our average patient was 56 and employed or retired following full-time employment (90%). 54% were married; 24% divorced, 18% widowed and 4% single. 10% had been widowed during the past 5 years and 50% had lost loved ones. 92% enjoyed good relationships with their families and 71% with their husbands. None of our patients kept the face-lift operation a secret. 20% told everyone they came in contact with about the operation and the same number told only members of their immediate families. The remaining 60% told their families and a few close friends.

Rhinoplasty Patients

Rhinoplasty is the other operation whose patient population has undergone intensive psychological study. As a rough rule, the older the date of publication of the study, the more disturbed the patients appear to be. Perhaps this is due to the decreasing social stigma and increasing 'respectability' of aesthetic surgery which has occurred over the past 30 years. Possibly it is due to a decreasing anti-aesthetic surgery bias on the part of the psychiatric investigators. It is certainly true that the extreme hostility toward aesthetic surgery that permeates the widely quoted 1956 paper by *Meerloo* [11] is not found in recent papers on the subject. Nonetheless, it is a fact that virtually all published studies suggest that rhinoplasty patients are more psychologically disturbed than the general population.

Linn and Goldman [19] studied rhinoplasty patients during the late 1940's. The great majority of these patients had psychiatric illnesses with diagnoses ranging from 'minor neurotic reactions' to 'overt schizophrenic psychoses'. Psychiatric diagnosis notwithstanding, most patients were found to have similar symptoms, which the researchers called the 'Psychiatric Syndrome of the Rhinoplasty Patient'. These patients are reclusive, shy, anxious in social situations and believe that others look down on them. They acquire mannerisms intended to hide from others what they regard as unfavorable views of their noses. Their manner is distracted, since they are unable to focus their attention for long on any situation because so much of their mental activity is 'distracted laterally', that is, constantly concerned with the nose. Others often interpret this distracted manner as an attitude of boredom, aloofness or unfriendliness, which, in turn, may lead to rejection by others – thus further reinforcing the patients' poor opinions of themselves. 'Almost all' of the patients in this study group were said to be afflicted with a 'severe generalized constriction of the ego'. This was reflected in constricted bodily movements, short attention span, difficulty concentrating and diminished capacity to develop warm relations with others.

We have no reason to doubt that the people studied by *Linn and Goldman* were typical rhinoplasty patients of the 1940's. We still see patients who seem to fall into the 'Psychiatric Syndrome' category, but not very often. The rhinoplasty patients of the 1980's, at least the young females, seem to be significantly healthier psychologically.

Older patients, particularly males, often seem to have considerably more psychopathology. Jacobson et al. [20] studied 20 men who sought facial aesthetic surgery for 'minimal defects', usually of the nose, sometimes of the upper lip or chin (these authors considered the nose, upper lip and chin to be a psychological, as well as an aesthetic surgical unit as do many plastic surgeons). Psychiatric diagnoses were assigned to all of the 18 men who agreed to psychiatric evaluation: 7 were psychotic, 4 were neurotic, and 7 had moderate to severe personality trait disorders. 9 of the 18 were operated upon and 5 of these had post-operative psychological disturbances. One made a serious suicide attempt.

Other studies also reflect considerable psychopathology in those seeking rhinoplasty. *Micheli-Pellegrini and Manfrida* [21] noted that 15 men in their study group of 65 showed more severe and more frequent psychological disturbances than the women. *Gibson and Connolly* [22] studied 194 British patients 10 years after rhinoplasty. 86 of them had rhinoplasties for nasal deformities due to disease or recent trauma. The remaining 118 had what, in the judgement of the surgeons, were purely aesthetic deformities. The surgeons who operated upon these patients were psychologically aware and knowledgeable in the art of patient selection. After 10 years only 8% of the disease and trauma group had a psychological disorder of any type and none was schizophrenic. In startling contrast, 38% of the aesthetic group had psychological disorders and 5 were schizophrenic. This study sharply reminds us of the fact that complaints of a physical deformity, especially a minor one that causes excessive concern, may be an early symptom of schizophrenia (dysmorphophobia, in the British usage).

Other studies of rhinoplasty patients also included control groups. *Hay* [23] and *Wright* [3] have reported controlled studies of rhinoplasty patients. 26 of *Hay's* 45 patients had personality disorders or psychoses. *Wright and Wright* also found that their rhinoplasty patients were more psychologically disturbed than a control group. The composite MMPI psychological profile of their rhinoplasty patients showed greater evidence of psychopathology than that of a control group having operations that were not aesthetic in nature. The rhinoplasty patients were generally intelligent, interesting, and likeable. Many were tense, restless, and mildly agitated. Their tendency was to be highly energetic, imaginative, enthusiastic, self-centered, and self-critical. They showed needs to dominate others and to act out, but were reluctant to take responsibility for their own behavior. They were not inclined to be open and kept their distance from others. Compared to the control group, the rhinoplasty patients were more restless, self-critical, and sensitive to the opinions of others. The most frequent psychological diagnosis was inadequate personality.

Blepharoplasty

Much less is known about patients seeking aesthetic surgery of the eyelid, blepharoplasty. A blepharoplasty is an operation designed to remove sagging eyelid skin and to reduce the puffiness of 'bags' due to 'herniated' fat pockets around the eyes. We are not aware of any reports in the literature of body image disturbances associated with this operation, although *Sheen* [24] has presented a paper on 'loss of identity' following blepharoplasty, and has alluded to it in a publication.

One of us (MKG) has interviewed and indirectly followed the clinical course of a woman in her mid-30's whose 'life was ruined' by a blepharoplasty. She described constant ruminations and obsessive thoughts about her eyes and the development of an intense anxiety that interfered with her ability to work. Following her operation she felt compelled to resign from a high-level executive position and to return to her parent's home to live a reclusive life. After the initial telephone interview, she was referred to another psychiatrist. She saw him only once, and subsequently saw two other psychiatrists. At one point she spent some time in a psychiatric hospital. Her psychiatrists assigned to her a variety of diagnoses: depressive reaction, severe obsessive-compulsive personality, and borderline personality.

Post-Operative Psychological Disturbances

Body Image Disturbances and Resultant Psychopathology

It is quite unusual for a restorative operation, such as a face-lift, to cause serious body image disturbances. Following a standard face-lift operation patients do not look 'different'. Their basic appearance is unchanged but they look younger and generally 'refreshed'. Friends commonly remark on how well they are looking but tend to attribute the improvement to a new hairstyle or a restful vacation. Thus, the average face-lift patient has little or no need to adjust psychologically to a sudden alteration in the size and shape of a body part with the attendant possibility of body image distortions.

Minor body image disturbances may occur after a standard face-lift. Most patients experience transient hypesthesia of the skin of the face and neck. The boundaries between self and non-self become blurred. Many patients, if asked, will describe this as a 'strange feeling'. It is disconcerting to try to sleep on a pillow which cannot be felt, or which is felt less distinctly than is usual. This rather odd experience may cause uneasiness, anxiety and sleeplessness. Rarely do such patients understand what it is that is keeping them awake. Often their insomnia can be cured by informing them of its cause and reassuring them that the diminished sensation will soon return to normal. Obviously, a simple explanation has no effect on the hypesthesia but it does reduce anxiety by assigning to it a 'normal' and expected cause.

Just as there are 'radical' and 'standard' face-lifts, there are restorative blepharoplasties and those which deliberately change the appearance by creating a new superior palpebral fold, as in the so-called 'oriental eyelid' operation. The authors have seen loss of identity ('I'm not myself anymore'. 'My friends say my eyes are bigger, smaller.') following both standard blepharoplasties and those of the 'type-changing' variety. Informal conversations with plastic surgeons lead us to believe that post-blepharo-plasty body image disturbances may be more common than is generally assumed.

Much has been written about the psychological significance of the nose and face in general but very little attention has been given to the eyes, at least in the literature dealing with the psychological aspects of plastic surgery. More investigation is needed. Everyone knows that eyes can express both character and emotion but it is less commonly understood that the anatomical variations that are perceived as mirroring internal characterological and psychoemotional tendencies reside not so much in the ocular globe itself but in periorbital structures such as the eyelids and associated muscles, the skin, the orbital rim, the lacrimal gland, and the brows, that is, those structures affected by the blepharoplasty and other ancillary plastic surgery operations. In time we may find that these structures – generally called 'the eye' – have as heavy a symbolic significance as the nose.

Body image disturbances have been reported with certain aesthetic plastic surgical interventions, presumably because of 'type changing' properties. For example, radical face-lift operations which include extensive fat removal from the face and neck may alter the appearance radically and give rise to distress.

Rhinoplasty has been reported far more frequently than other aesthetic facial surgical procedures to be associated with psychiatric disturbances. *Knorr* [25] described 9 women (ages 26–64) who experienced a loss of identity of 'the old self' following rhinoplasty. A common theme was their belief that 'too much had been done' resulting in an undesirably drastic change in appearance. A number of these women had considerable medical histories and showed an insatiable need for further corrective surgery which rarely satisfied them or restored their lost identities. Body image disturbances of such intensity are rare; but similar, milder, time-limited reactions are not particularly uncommon while patients are becoming accustomed to their new appearances. Uneasiness or anxiety about changes in the body should not be confused with pleasure or displeasure with the physical results of an operation. Patients may be very unhappy about their appearance after an operation and have no evidence of body image disturbances while others with relatively severe body image disturbances may be delighted with the surgical outcome. Needless to say, dissatisfaction may coexist with body image disturbances and vice versa. In any case, the surgeon or psychiatrist needs to clarify the situation for both clinician and patient. Only in this way can the appropriate interventions be made: in certain cases education of the patient about body image disturbances may be in order while in others the surgeon may need to consider surgical revision.

Psychosis after Aesthetic Facial Surgery

Psychotic reactions are rarely precipitated by aesthetic facial surgery but when this catastrophe does occur, the operative procedure most frequently implicated is rhinoplasty. In all the cases known to us of plastic surgeons murdered by their patients in the past 30 years, the assailants have all had rhinoplasties.

Druss [26] described a Caucasian woman who felt that her rhinoplasty had made her look negroid. A long-standing psychotic delusion that her father (whom she had never seen) was black was the psychological basis for her post-operative delusion. We [10] have written about a woman whose rhinoplasty was followed by psychotic decompensation. She repeatedly demanded that the surgeon re-operate on her nose. Believing that her physical result was the best that he could achieve, the surgeon refused. Her delusions intensified and one morning he received a call from the University emergency department where she was being resuscitated following attempted suicide. Perhaps because of the inadequate pre-operative screening interview, the surgeon was unaware that she had the delusion that bad odors emanated from her nose. The patient's psychiatrist had been well aware of this, but the surgeon failed to talk to him. As a result of this operation on a body part directly involved in a delusional system, a relatively stable chronic schizophrenic regressed to a deeper psychotic state. Both of these patients had psychotic delusions about their noses, were chronic schizophrenics, and as a result of destabilizing operations became floridly psychotic.

The nose has been reported [27] to have sexual symbolism for both men and women. Post-operative disturbances related to the sexual symbolism of the nose, however, have been reported much more frequently in men. A man's feelings about his nose can conceal intense anxieties about his sexual identity and masculinity. One example of the nose-penis 'equation' and its potential for provoking psychological disturbance is represented by the case of a man who became psychotic following a rhinoplasty. His unconscious conflicts about his sexual identity had become displaced onto concerns about the size and shape of his nose. Post-operatively, the real psychological issues remained unresolved. He became paranoid and developed the delusion that his nose was undergoing a slow necrotic process and would eventually disappear.

Post-Operative Depression

Depression is not a single entity but encompasses: major depressive disorder; bipolar affective disorder, depressed; atypical depressive disorder; adult adjustment reaction with depressive features; and, less formally, 'the blues' and 'feeling down'. These differentiations must be kept clearly in mind when one is trying to understand post-operative depression. A few years ago we decided to undertake a psychological study of 50 female face-lift patients [15]. We were stimulated to do so in part by the clinical impression of many plastic surgeons that post-operative depression was more common following face-lift than any other operation. The findings of our study unmistakably underscored the fact that a number of variables, including timing, intensity and etiology, must be considered in order to understand post-operative depression. In view of the plastic surgeons' impressions, it is interesting to note that the incidence of significant depressive symptoms following face-lifts (approximately 30%) was very similar to that reported years ago by *Lindemann* [28] in patients undergoing major abdominal surgery.

Some indication of depression was noted in 54% of our patients. In 24% transient episodes of 'the blues' or feeling 'down' occurred, either immediately after the operation of 2–3 weeks later. More intense and persistent symptoms of depression (insomnia, psychomotor retardation, and mild anorexia) were seen in 30%, but none became psychotically depressed or suicidal. We looked for predictors of post-operative depression and found that characterological patterns and the pre-operative presence of depressive symptoms were a more accurate prediction than such factors as: psychological reactions to body change, pleasure or displeasure with the operative result, or unrealistic or secret motivations. Indeed more than half of the patients revealed unrealistic or secret motivations to the research psychiatrist (but not to the surgeon). Some patients did not become consciously aware of these motivations until after the operation, when their secret desires failed to materialize.

Only 2 of the women with these unrealistic or secret motivations became depressed. Both were struggling with mid-life crises [29]. After their operations both looked but did not feel younger, and the denial which they had been dealing with in their mid-life crises dissolved. One of the two, a widow, experienced a dawning realization of her loneliness and fear. Pre-operatively she had denied any wish for a permanent relationship and said that she regarded her husband's death not as a loss rather as a gain of a long desired sense of freedom. The other woman, whose husband had recently retired, had been trying to deny her growing realization that their relationship was empty and her concerns about how to deal with this insight. She found that her new, youthful appearance not only failed to remedy this basic problem but brought it into clear focus.

In the immediate post-operative period, the women who became transiently depressed or agitated were aggressive, active and assertive. Characteristically, they were independent and self-reliant. The inactivity and dependence upon others enforced by convalescence were difficult for them to deal with. As their energy returned and physical restrictions imposed by the operation were lifted, one could see their depressive symptoms fade away. This early period was particularly trying for some older women who found that their strength did not return as rapidly as it had in the past.

Those who developed transient depressions 2 or 3 weeks post-operatively had personalities of a very different type. These were women with strong needs to be cared for and nurtured. Usually their dependency needs were met by nurturing people with whom they surrounded themselves. But as bandages and stitches disappeared and bruises faded, the nurturing wells began to run dry and they found themselves thrown on their own resources. This, we believe, accounted for the timing of their depressive reactions.

There is little doubt that the most common antecedent of post-operative depression is a pre-existing depressive state. Sometimes this pre-existing depression is obvious; a patient will burst into tears when a surgeon asks, 'How are things going?'. In other cases it may be unconsciously denied or masked by the secret hope that the operation will alter some unalterable life stress. In these instances depressive symptoms may not be transient and should be treated appropriately as any other depression would be treated.

Post-Operative Acting Out

Occasionally even the most favorable changes resulting from an aesthetic operation will precipitate self-destructive behavior patterns. The ugly duckling suddenly transformed into a lovely swan will find herself facing new and unfamiliar experiences. Those who are shy and inhibited because of their appearance tend to pass through adolescence like shadows, blending into the background of that turbulent time, and participating in it as little as possible.

Post-operatively – and this applies particularly to some young rhinoplasty patients – they find themselves suddenly attractive, with new self-confidence and self-esteem, and begin to behave more assertively. They find that they must learn to deal with the changed response of others to their new, more confident and assertive selves.

This much desired surgical change, however, can cause problems. Adolescence is a time of trial and error, of testing limits, of learning to deal with one's emerging sexuality, of magical hopes and dreams, and of success and rejection. Those who have not passed through this crucible and are suddenly plunged into something very like it, at an accelerated rate and without a supporting peer group, may find themselves 'in over their heads'. Then they have to cope with a variety of new impulses and temptations. Psychotherapy can often be very helpful in consolidating their gains in a constructive fashion.

Psychological Improvement

Surgical alterations in the size and shape of the nose or the removal of sagging skin can often produce surprisingly positive psychological results. *Wright and Wright* [3] studied the pre-operative and post-operative MMPI profiles of a group of rhinoplasty patients. Pre-operatively their profiles were significantly elevated on the psychopathic deviant-manic scales as compared to the MMPI profiles of a group of patients having non-aesthetic operations. The non-aesthetic patients were 'less restless, self critical, and sensitive to the opinions of others'. The psychopathic deviant scale was also lower in the control group. The rhinoplasty patients were re-evaluated 18–24 months after their operations. While these patients did not undergo major personality changes, they did show improvement in self-concept, a decrease in aggressive impulses, and less somatization. The mild agitation/depressed pattern noted pre-operatively disappeared and energy and activity levels moved closer to the normal range. They also seemed more self-confident in social situations and more adept in establishing, maintaining, and enjoying relationships.

A survey which we [10] carried out confirms the psychological benefits of rhinoplasty as well as its psychological hazards in poorly selected patients. This group of rhinoplasty patients was a rather special one. All of them were under treatment by psychoanalysts and the information was obtained by interviewing the psychoanalysts rather than the patients themselves. 25 out of 100 psychoanalysts surveyed provided us with information about 27 rhinoplasty patients, 2 of whom began treatment as a result of the psychological effects of a recent rhinoplasty. Post-operatively 6 of the group were worsened psychologically, 9 showed no psychological change, and 12 were improved psychologically.

In many instances the psychological improvement came as a genuine surprise to the psychoanalyst who, in some cases 'saw nothing wrong' with the patient's nose and could not comprehend how such a minimal physical alteration could be of such importance. In other cases these therapists feared that the patient's concerns about the nose represented a displacement of intrapsychic conflicts. One patient, for example, had intense conflicts about his sexual identity. His psychiatrist feared that this anxiety over his masculinity and sexuality had been displaced to his nose, and that an operation on this highly symbolic structure would intensify these conflicts. Because this man had been able to separate his concerns about his sexuality from his dislike of his nose, his post-operative reaction was entirely positive. He became less self-conscious about his appearance and his self-confidence increased. He began to take a number of positive steps in his life that previously he had only been able to ruminate about.

Rather surprisingly, some of the psychoanalysts who participated in this survey confessed that they were not familiar with the concept that a surgical change in the body could result in anything other than a psychological disruptive effect. The positive as well as the negative psychological effects of aesthetic plastic surgery need wider dissemination in the psychiatric community.

Two facts came out of this study. The first is that what appears to be a 'minimal defect' of someone else's nose can be and often is strongly disliked by the individual to whom the nose belongs. Others cannot judge the importance of a rhinoplasty to a patient simply by looking at the nose. Small improvements in the size or contour may result in great psychological improvement, while changes that seem strikingly good to others may result in no benefit to the patient. The second conclusion that we drew from our survey is that the pre-operative existence of conflicts about sexual identity is not predictive of post-operative psychological disturbance. Those who are aware of these intrapsychic conflicts and do not confuse them with their dislike of their noses can have a very good psychological outcome when the desired result is achieved surgically. It is only when the intrapsychic conflicts have been displaced onto the nose and confused with the desire for a new nose that disaster can be expected.

Similar psychological improvement was observed in some patients in our study of face-lift patients [15]. Certain patients were found pre-operatively to have clinical evidence of depression, elevated Beck Depression Inventory Scales [30] and elevated MMPI depression scales. In the immediate post-operative period their depressive symptoms became more severe, but at 6 months a lifting of the pre-operative level of depression was noted. These women also reported increased feelings of self-esteem and self-confidence. Apparently, the external, cutaneous manifestations of aging intensified life-long feelings of inadequacy and depression.

The patients who improved psychologically differed from a small group whose expressed concerns about facial aging changes actually masked their mid-life concerns about aging, dependence, and the changing patterns of life associated with retirement or widowhood. As will be clear at this point, the face-lift operation could not have any real effect on these things. Post-operatively their emotional disturbances intensified rather than decreased.

14 of the women in the study described a post-operative increase in their self-esteem, new-found self-confidence and the ability to be more assertive. Women whose self-consciousness about their aging appearance had inhibited advancement in their careers described a post-operative change in this attitude. They were more confident that their capabilities were respected. They volunteered for increasingly difficult tasks and requested assignments to important committees. One woman stated: 'I'm trying in all the ways I know to get the senior executive position I want. Before the operation, I didn't have the courage. Even if I don't get the the job I won't mind as much as before, knowing I've given it my all.' A major predictor for this type of improvement was the pre-operatively expressed desire that the operation would improve self-image.

A surprising finding in the study was the correlation of a positive psychological outcome with the presence of relatively higher scores on the MMPI paranoia scale. Several patients believed that they were stigmatized and rejected because of their haggard appearance. As a result of this belief, they had withdrawn from social contacts and were leading quite isolated lives. After the operation, whatever unacceptable emotions that they believed were previously revealed by their 'haggard' look (anger, resentment, grief, etc.) were masked by the refreshed appearance. The vicious cycle of fear and rejection leading to isolation was interrupted and with it there was an opportunity to test the reality of the reactions of others. In several instances this led to greatly improved relationships.

Self-consciousness about appearance can strongly affect self-confidence and self-esteem. Pleasure with the result of an aesthetic operation may diminish self-consciousness and increase self-confidence. An aesthetic surgery patient's comment about the face-lift operation that, 'I never think about my face anymore' is usually a very positive sign. It reflects the fact that previous concerns about appearance are no longer a consideration. Whatever roadblock those feelings created has been removed and the patient can get on with the business of living.

The Psychiatrist as Consultant

When an ICU nurse calls a psychiatrist at two in the morning about a post-operative coronary artery bypass patient with normal blood chemistries and electrolytes who is agitated, confused and hallucinating, the reason for the consultation will be apparent and the psychiatrist may see no need to telephone the referring physician, at least at that time.

The situation may be considerably more enigmatic when a plastic surgeon refers a patient, and even more so when a patient calls saying he has been referred by a plastic surgeon. Before seeing such a patient, it is imperative that the psychiatrist talk to the surgeon to find out: why the surgeon has referred the patient, what are the important issues for exploration and what the patient has been told about the reason for the referral. While this advice may sound (and be) simplistic, it is based on the certain knowledge that many plastic surgeons are extremely uncomfortable about making a psychiatric referral and may be quite maladroit in doing so. Some may even 'soften the blow' of the referral by neglecting to mention that the consultant is a psychiatrist. Instead something may be muttered about 'an expert', or 'nerve doctor', or 'counselor'. Furthermore, the plastic surgeon may not have a very clear idea as to the reason for the referral and may not know exactly how the psychiatrist can help. A conversation with the plastic surgeon – who may never have referred a patient to a psychiatrist before and may be doing so in this instance as a last 'end of the rope' gesture – about the various ways in which a psychiatric consultation can be useful, allows the plastic surgeon to understand the multiple uses of consultation psychiatry. Consequently, if the patient or anyone other than the plastic surgeon telephones to make an appointment for such a consultation, the psychiatrist should be sure to talk directly with the surgeon. This will help to clarify the questions that have been raised, and the reasons that precipitated the request for psychiatric referral.

Reasons for Referral

Most commonly, perhaps, the plastic surgeon will be trying to decide whether a patient is emotionally suitable for (will not be harmed psychologically by) an operation. Is the patient psychotic? Is there a delusion involving the body part to be operated upon? The surgeon will be concerned as to whether the patient is so unstable emotionally as to be unable to deal with the stress of *any* elective operation. Does the operation have a special, unconscious, symbolic meaning for the patient? Is this, for instance, a man who is troubled by questions about his masculine identity, for whom a rhinoplasty may trigger even more intense feelings of inadequacy? Or is this a man with similar concerns yet who recognizes his intrapsychic conflicts, does not confuse them with feelings of dissatisfaction with his nose and may do quite well after a nasal operation?

At other times the surgeon may recognize psychological problems but feels that the patient can be helped surgically if rapport is established pre-operatively with a psychiatrist who can be available for support and treatment during the post-operative period.

Rarely, an enlightened plastic surgeon may refer a young patient who has had a good surgical result but needs help in consolidating the gains resulting from the ugly duckling to swan transformation. As psychiatrists achieve better liaison with plastic surgeons, this kind of referral should become more common.

Sometimes a patient may be referred for psychiatric treatment when the surgeon has no intention of operating on an obviously psychotic patient. In some instances psychologically unsophisticated surgeons may send a patient for 'clearance' for surgery, in the same way they might send a patient to an internist or cardiologist. Unfortunately, there are no psychiatric EKGs and treadmill tests to give these surgeons the answer they want. The psychiatrist's responsibility is heavy in such cases and discussion with the surgeon is crucial.

When the patient is specifically referred to determine emotional suitability for surgery, the psychiatrist needs to be certain that the patient understands this and that the psychiatrist will of necessity be communicating with the plastic surgeon. This does not mean that the psychiatrist will not keep privacy issues in mind, but the patient needs to be clear about the need for an exchange of information and authorize the release of that information which is necessary for optimal medical care.

Relevant Clinical Questions

Before the psychiatrist can make an accurate assessment of the patient's psychological fitness for a given operation, the specifics of that operation must be known. How long does it take? General or local anesthesia? Is it a restorative operation (like a face-lift) or is it a type-changing procedure that makes a patient look strikingly different and will involve body image changes, distortions, or disturbances? What will be the quality of the physical results? Does the surgeon consider the patient a poor, fair, good or excellent physical candidate for the operation? Will there be significant sensory changes – numbness of the face or nipples for example – and if so, how long will such changes last? What are the risks of the procedure?

In an interview with a prospective plastic surgery patient, certain specific areas need to be addressed, beyond those that ordinarily enable the psychiatrist to arrive at a diagnostic formulation. How long has the patient been unhappy with the body part in question? The average rhinoplasty patient will say that he/she has disliked the nose 'forever' or 'as long as I can remember'. Adolescent teasing and resulting self-consciousness explain this. The sudden emergence or dissatisfaction with a more-or-less unchanging body part (ear, nose or chin for example) at the age of 35 should raise the question 'why now?'. To some extent this holds for those requesting aesthetic surgery for facial aging changes. The widow whose answer to 'why now?' is that she never thought about her gradually aging appearance until her husband's death may be giving a quite logical explanation for her wish for a face-lift. Another woman's sudden desire for a face-lift may reflect her wish to recapture the attention of her straying husband. The face-lift operation can do some psychologically useful things, but it has never been shown to be the means of saving a dying marriage.

Patients referred because they are experiencing life crises present an interesting problem. Some plastic surgeons believe that all such patients should have their operation deferred for some arbitrary length of time, commonly six months. This policy may not always be in the patient's best interest.

The psychiatrist can help here by determining whether the request for an operation is a positive adaptive step, representing an attempt at resolution, or whether it is a straw-grasping effort to deny the underlying problem.

One question that the psychiatrist should always have in mind concerns the symbolic meaning of the body part to be altered. In aesthetic surgery of the face, this is particularly true of the nose. Is sudden late-blooming concern with the nose an early symptom of schizophrenia? Is the patient requesting a rhinoplasty: to eliminate a bump or narrow the tip, to eliminate a bad odor imagined to be emanating from the nose, or because of fears of sexual inadequacy?

Familial attitudes and characteristics are important in all aesthetic surgery, in terms of support for or hostility toward the proposed operation. Positive and negative 'feedback' from family members can greatly influence a patient's satisfaction with an aesthetic operation. Such attitudes and characteristics are particularly important in rhinoplasty patients. Does the patient's nose resemble that of a family member? Is that family member loved or hated? Is the patient's nose characteristic or uncharacteristic of 'the family nose'? Does the patient truly understand that post-operatively he may no longer resemble his mother or father? Will the patient be able to cope with this loss? Is the patient's nose considered by the patient and family to be an ethnic stereotype – a 'typical' Jewish, Armenian, or Italian nose? If so, will changing this 'typical' nose be perceived by the family as an attempt to reject a cherished heritage? Have other members of the family had a similar operation? How do they regard the results of their operations?

These are some of the questions that need to be asked in order to ascertain whether a particular patient will be psychologically harmed by a given operation. If what the surgeon wants from a psychiatric consultation can be capsulized in a single question, it is this: 'Will my patient be made worse psychologically by the proposed operation?' If the psychiatrist feels that psychological improvement may occur, all the better. But the purpose of a psychiatric consultation is not to select only those who will obtain detectable psychological improvement. Many patients derive genuine pleasure and satisfaction from aesthetic operations without showing any psychological changes. The most reassuring and reliable responses from patients are those that indicate that their motivations for surgery are internalized, related to self-image and self-esteem. Motives which involve the hoped-for effect of the operation on others are less often realizable and may reflect magical thinking.

Post-Operative Psychiatric Care

Transient Psychological Problems

Transient psychological problems are not uncommon following facial aesthetic surgical procedures. When the psychiatrist is familiar with these, the kind of understanding and reassurance that facilitates their resolution can be provided. Many patients who seek aesthetic surgery are assertive and active and may feel anxious and 'blue' immediately after an operation. The enforced inactivity and confinement interferes with the use of their usual coping mechanisms. Other, more passive-dependent patients may enjoy the concern and care of others in the immediate post-operative period and then become depressed about 2 weeks after the operation, when the support of others diminishes and they find themselves thrown on their own resources. These depressive reactions tend to resolve spontaneously and ordinarily require only supportive care.

Body image disturbances also usually resolve with time [31]. It takes a while to adjust psychologically to being a new size and shape. Patients who do not understand the 'normality' of feelings and sensations that accompany body image changes may become panicky and anxious about sudden uncertainties about where they begin and end. Other body image disturbances may be caused by temporary alterations in sensation. The transient diminution in sensation that regularly follows the face-lift operation may sometimes cause insomnia. In such instances sleeplessness is not necessarily due to post-operative depression but to the 'funny' feeling of not knowing precisely where one's cheek ends and the pillow begins. Recognition of the problem and defining its cause for the patient may relieve the anxiety and cure the insomnia.

Long Term Psychological Problems

Occasionally, a pre-existing, severe depressive reaction may be unmasked by an aesthetic facial operation and should be treated as any other depressive reaction.

Psychotic decompensation is rare but does occur. From the data available, it appears to be more common following rhinoplasty than any other aesthetic facial operation. Inferences as to the reason for this may be drawn from the special psychological significance of the nose and the studies showing the rhinoplasty population to be more disturbed than people in general.

Problems with Social Adjustment

Psychiatrists may be asked to see post-operative plastic surgery patients who are having difficulties with social adjustment. A patient typifying this group would be a once-shy, withdrawn, and socially-inept woman in her 20's who, following a rhinoplasty, becomes attractive and self-confident and begins to behave so as to call more attention to herself by changing her hairstyle, buying stylish clothes, and accepting previously-declined or never-before-offered invitations. On the surface these adaptive changes may seem entirely positive but inside her 25 year old self, she may be experiencing all the anxieties and torments of the adolescence she never really had, without the support of an adolescent peer-group with which to relate, discuss, share experiences, and talk about appropriate responses. Her life may become progressively more chaotic and this may lead her to seek or agree to treatment. Recognition of the factors which precipitate such changes will enable the psychiatrist to understand why this disturbance should appear at this particular time and to help her to work through her problems, almost as one would work with an adolescent trying to deal with an identity crisis.

Defining the question to be asked, learning the post-operative danger signals as well as the positive and negative pre-operative indicators, and becoming more knowledgeable about post-operative psychological stress will help to make the psychiatrist a useful member of the surgical team. It may also open some doors which will lead to further learning and perhaps research about psychological mind-body interactions.

References

1   Obendorf, C.P.: Submucous resection as a castration symbol. Int. J. Psychoanal. *10:* 228 (1929).
2   Hill, G.; Silver, A.J.: Psychodynamic and esthetic motivation for plastic surgery. Psychosom. Med. *12:* 345 (1950).
3   Wright, M.R.; Wright, W.K.: A psychological study of patients undergoing cosmetic surgery. Arch. Otolaryngol. *101:* 125 (1975).
4   Freud, S.: The Ego and the Id. pp. 26 (Hogarth Press, London 1927).
5   McDevitt, J.G.; Settlage, K.F.: Separation Individuation: Essays in Honor of Margaret Mahler. (International University Press, New York 1971).
6   Mahler, S.M.; McDevitt, J.B.: Thoughts on the emergence of the sense of self, with particular emphasis on the body self. J. Am. Psychoanal. Ass. *30:* 837 (1982).
7   Kohut, H.; Wolf, E.: The disorders of the self and their treatment: an outline. Int. J. Psychoanal. *59:* 413–425 (1978).

8   Erikson, E.: Eight stages of man; in Erikson, E., Childhood and Society, pp. 219–234 (W.W. Norton & Co., New York 1950).

9   Bercleid, E.; Walster, E.: Beauty and the best. Psychol. Today. *5:* March (1972).

10 Goin, M.D.; Goin, J.M.: Changing the Body: Psychological Effects of Plastic Surgery, Chapter 13 (Williams and Wilkins, Baltimore, 1981).

11 Meerloo, J.A.M.: The fate of one's face. Psychiatr. Q. *30:* 31 (1956).

12 Buhler, C.: The curve of life as studied in biographies. J. Appl. Psychol. *19:* 405 (1935).

13 Buhler, C.: Maturation and motivation. Personality *1:* 18 (1951).

14 Goin, M.D.; Burgoyne, R.W.; Goin, J.M.: Face-lift operation: The patient's secret motivations and reactions to 'Informed Consent'. Plast. Reconstr. Surg. *58:* 273 (1976).

15 Goin, M.K.; Burgoyne, R.W.; Goin, J.M.; Staples, F.R.: A prospective psychological study of 50 female face-lift patients. Plast. Reconstr. Surg. *65:* 436 (1980).

16 Webb, W.L., Jr.; Slaughter, R.; Meyer, E.; Edgerton, M.: Mechanism of psychosocial adjustment in patients seeking 'face-lift' operations. Psychosom. Med. *27:* 83 (1965).

17 Baker, T.J.: Patient selection and psychological evaluation. Clin. Plast. Surg. *5:* 3 (1978).

18 Baker, T.J.; Gordon, H.L.; Mosienko, R.: Rhytidectomy: A statistical analysis. Plast. Reconstr. Surg *59:* 24 (1977).

19 Linn, L.; Goldman, I.B.: Psychiatric observations concerning rhinoplasty. Psychosom. Med. *11:* 307 (1949).

20 Jacobson, W.; Edgerton, M.; Meyer, E.; Canter, A.; Slaughter, R.: Psychiatric evaluation of male patients seeking cosmetic surgery. Plast. Reconstr. Surg. *26:* 356 (1960).

21 Micheli-Pellegrini, V.; Manfrida, G.M.: Rhinoplasty and its psychological implications: Applied psychology observations in aesthetic surgery. Aesthet. Plast. Surg. *3:* 229 (1979).

22 Gibson, M.; Connolly, F.H.: The incidence of schizophrenia and severe psychological disorders in patients 10 years after cosmetic rhinoplasty. Br. J. Plast. Surg. *28:* 125 (1978).

23 Hay, G.G.: Psychiatric aspects of cosmetic nasal operations. Br. J. Psychiatry *116:* 85 (1970).

24 Sheen, J.H.: Supratarsal fixation in upper blepharoplasty; in Goulian, D.; Courtiss, E.H. eds., Symposium on surgery of the aging face, Chapter 15 (C.V. Mosby Co., St. Louis, 1978).

25 Knorr, N.J.: Feminine loss of identity in rhinoplasty. Arch. Otolaryngol. *96:* 11 (1972).

26 Druss, R.G.; Symonds, F.C.; Crickelair, G.L.: The problem of somatic delusions in patients seeking cosmetic surgery. Plast. Reconstr. Surg. *46:* 246 (1971).

27 Book, H.E.: Sexual implications of the nose. Compr. Psychiatry *12:* 450 (1971).

28 Lindemann, E.: Observations on psychiatric sequelae to surgical operations in women. Am. J. Psychiatr. *98:* 132 (1941).

29 Jaques, E.: Death and mid-life crisis. Int. J. of Psychoanal. *46:* 502–514 (1965).

30 The Beck Depression Scale may be obtained at Aaron T. Beck, M.D., Center for Cognitive Therapy, 133 South 36th Street, Room 602, Philadelphia, Pa. 19104.

31 Goin, J.M.; Goin, M.K.: Changing the Body: Psychological Effects of Plastic Surgery, Chapter 7 (Williams and Wilkins, Baltimore 1981).

Marcia Kraft Goin, MD, PhD, University of Southern California, School of Medicine, Los Angeles, CA 90005 (USA)

Adv. psychosom. Med., vol. 15, pp. 109–123 (Karger, Basel 1986)

Psychiatric Sequelae Following Surgical Treatment of Breast Cancer

Jimmie C. Holland, Ellen Jacobs

Cornell University Medical College and Psychiatry Service, Memorial Sloan-Kettering Cancer Center, New York, N.Y., USA

Today, women who undergo mastectomy are medically sophisticated. The choice of mastectomy has often been made after thoughtful consideration of lumpectomy and radiation. Treatment options are mandated by law in some states. After mastectomy, women are told the type, extent and size of the cancer which was removed; they are told of the presence, number and site of positive axillary nodes. The psychological impact on loss of a meaningful body part is compounded by the direct confrontation with the threat to life and uncertainty about the future. This dual stress has been noted to have a major psychological impact on women over the last 30 years [1]. The newer practice of full disclosure and participation in decision-making, however, has increased the stress at the early stage of diagnosis and treatment decision.

The standard initial treatment for breast cancer, radical surgical removal, remained the same until the last decade. Some of the earliest major studies of post-mastectomy psychological adjustment were carried out at Memorial Sloan-Kettering Cancer Center in the early 1950's by the *Sutherland group* [2]. They found that women experienced varying degrees of depression, anxiety and anger. Their everyday life patterns were disrupted, with major impact on self-esteem and sexual function. Fear regarding recurrence of cancer, unsightly lymphedema of the arm and distortion of the chest wall after radical mastectomy were painful aspects of reality.

The magnitude of problems associated with breast cancer is still great. It affects one in 11 women. A sharp increase in the rates for both black and white women has occurred over the last 20 years. In 1985, as many as 119,000 women and their families per year now face this physical and psychological stress [3]. Such numbers underscore the need for a clear understanding of those factors which lead to a good psychological adaptation as well as to those which increase psychiatric morbidity. While many reports have described successful adaptation, despite emotional distress, other women who are distressed have been reluctant to acknowledge problems, creating a pretense of well-being [4–6]. Medical personnel often are not informed of emotional distress by the patient unless they inquire directly about it [7]. Patients themselves often pay a high emotional price for 'looking good' and not complaining.

The current decade has seen earlier detection of breast cancer, less extensive surgery, better plastic reconstructive procedures, and a new era of women participating in decisions about their own treatment, particularly the more frequent request for a two-stage procedure which separates biopsy from mastectomy. Some 'old' psychological problems have been replaced by 'new' ones which, while different, are no less stressful.

Historical Perspective

Perhaps no other tumor site has undergone more drastic and rapid change in its surgical management than breast cancer in the past decade. For well over 50 years, the radical mastectomy was the accepted procedure for operable breast cancer. Devised by *Charles Moore* in England well over a century ago, it was quickly adopted by *Halstead and Willy Meyer* in the United States (8). Following *Halstead's* report in 1898, the procedure quickly became the standard treatment for breast cancer [9]. Radical mastectomy involves an *en bloc* dissection of the entire breast and skin, together with the pectoralis major and minor muscles and the contents of the axilla. Some surgeons, in an effort to remove all possible tumor cells, developed the 'extended radical' which included dissection of the internal mammary lymphatic chain. The standard and extended radical procedure routinely produced a lymphedematous arm with limited function and a deformed 'washboard' chest wall of exposed rib structure at the operative site. Those women experienced significant physical limitations of function in their work and family roles. They had few social or psychological supports available to them beyond those in their own families. Breast surgery was rarely discussed with others since it was a subject involving taboos associated both with cancer and with the breast as a sexual organ.

In the early 1970's, debates began to occur about the efficacy of less extensive breast surgery. A heated dialogue is chronicled in the JAMA in 1974 between *Crile*, who reported 10 year equal survival with partial (modified) radical mastectomy, and *Haagenson and Anglem*, who advocated continued use of the radical mastectomy [10]. *Fisher* has brought a more rational approach to this debate by conducting a series of controlled randomized clinical trials to obtain data on efficacy of treatment choices, as Chairman of the National Surgical Adjuvant Breast Project (NSABP) [11].

Fisher stated that there are two aims in the management of primary breast cancer: to achieve a disease-free life, and to obtain the best possible cosmesis without compromising chance for cure. The 'state of the art' in the past decade has moved from an era in which the unequivocal standard treatment was radical mastectomy, with or without radiation, to a period of admitted therapeutic uncertainty which includes less radical surgery and the use of radiation and chemotherapy. Both eras have resulted in significant (but quite different) psychological problems for women faced with treatment of this most common female cancer.

Several major factors have contributed to the change: 1) new insights into the disease as a systemic one; 2) better treatment of advanced disease, resulting in principles of treatment for lesser degrees of disease; 3) improvement of survival by use of systems approach to treatment; and 4) the use of randomized clinical trials to determine the best treatment. Surgery had been based solely upon anatomic considerations, with cure being assumed to be related to removing 'the last cell', even with local and regional spread, by *en bloc* dissection. Despite improved techniques, however survival did not improve. Therefore, a reconsideration of treatment approach was undertaken, with the rational aim of surgery to reduce the viable tumor cells to a number that could be destroyed by host immunologic factors, chemotherapeutic agents or both [11].

Current Treatment Modalities

Current treatment for breast cancer commonly employs one or more of the procedures below. It is immediately clear that one cannot any longer assume that the same psychological sequelae reported in women who received the *Halstead* radical mastectomy will be seen in women who experience far less extensive procedures. The less extensive operation is associated with far better physical function, less extensive chest deformity and the opportunity – for the first time – for breast reconstruction.

1. *Modified radical mastectomy.* In this most common procedure, the breast is entirely removed with axillary dissection, but the pectoralis major, and often minor, muscles are spared. The functional result is greatly improved.

2. *Total (Simple) mastectomy.* The entire breast is removed but the pectoralis muscle and axilla are left intact.

3. *Segmental resection (lumpectomy).* The tumor is removed and the adjacent section of breast. This is done for tumors under 3 centimeters; it may or may not be accompanied by axillary dissection [12].

4. *Primary radiation.* Today, some physicians advocate radiation treatment alone for small lesions under 2 cm. Survival data are still early but it appears that mortality is only slightly less than with surgical resection; some European series report no difference in survival [13].

5. *Plastic reconstruction.* Any of the above procedures may be combined with immediate or delayed breast reconstructive procedures, using a plastic breast implant [14–16]. Plastic surgery following mastectomy has become far better accepted by breast and general surgeons who now usually discuss the option with women.

6. *Prophylactic mastectomy.* Breast Self-Examination (BSE) and mammography are recommended as useful in early detection of breast cancer, particularly in women at high risk [17–19]. High genetic risk or fibrocystic disease raises the question of prophylactic mastectomy as a viable treatment option [20]. Some patients make this request in an attempt to alleviate anxiety about 'waiting' to develop a tumor. The decision requires careful consideration of the medical, surgical and psychological aspects.

Current Sociocultural Climate

Major changes have also occurred in the sociocultural context which continuously interact with the medical and surgical advances; each impacts on the other. An abrupt change in attitude occurred in the fall of 1975, when both *Betty Ford's and Happy Rockefeller's* diagnosis of breast cancer, type of treatment and extent of disease were made public. Prior to that, information given to the patient was generally kept to a minimum and medical facts were less openly discussed, both between doctors and patient, and between a patient and her family and friends. Following the *Ford and Rockefeller* disclosures, done with remarkable candor, women began to call surgeons to inquire about their diagnosis (frequently not revealed before) and how many positive axillary nodes they had. Women also began an increasingly active movement to participate in decisions about their medical care in general and breast cancer in particular [20, 21]. Self-help groups, similar to Reach-for-Recovery, were begun. Such groups have gained increasingly free access to the medical establishment, providing a new service and a collective voice for women who want to ask questions and effect changes in decision making. All American Cancer Society divisions, as well as the National Office, have available and easily accessible information.

The medical and sociocultural climate in which a woman now has breast cancer is thus very different from that of 10 to 20 years ago. The events that characterize the clinical course of the disease and the parallel psychological reactions will be reviewed in light of the changes that have been described.

Patients' Concerns about Clinical Issues

Anxiety about the possibility of breast cancer is aroused as soon as a woman suspects or finds a lump in her breast [22]. Her decision to seek medical attention at that time is dependent upon a number of psychological and social factors, including her knowledge of, and attitude towards, medical care and cancer; her feelings about her breasts; and previous and current patterns of coping with stress, particularly the use of denial as a defense against anxiety which can contribute to delay [23].

Women today are better informed about the usefulness of mammography and the value of information and fears about early detection [24], but they are also cautious in view of possible effects of exposure to excessive radiation [25]. Awareness of the need for screening, even in the absence of early symptoms, stimulates fears of cancer and concerns of a life-threatening disease requiring surgery [26].

Watching and Waiting

Once a woman is examined, the decision is made to either 'watch and wait' or to biopsy the suspicious area either by needle biopsy or excision under anesthesia. Some women are simply too fearful to watch and wait; often the conviction that 'something is really wrong' proves poignantly to be the case. Others may deny the potential seriousness of the symptom, interpret the physician's 'delay' as absence of concern and be lost to follow up.

Decision for biopsy in the past carried with it the acceptance of biopsy under anesthesia with permission given the surgeon to do the mastectomy as well if the biopsy was found to be positive on frozen section. This 'one stage' procedure has been replaced, in recent years, by the 'two stage' approach, performing a biopsy done in an ambulatory surgical setting under local anesthesia. If positive, the second stage with mastectomy is then anticipated and the patient can prepare for absence from home and loss of a breast. During this period of anticipation, *Katz* et al. found that women who used denial and repression, and those who were fatalistic, stoic or who used prayer and faith were least visibly distressed and showed less stress activation of the hypothalamic-pituitary-adrenal axis (HPA). They were more likely, however, to delay longer in coming in. Conversely, women who showed more despair, anger and distress had activation of the HPA [27]. This is clearly a period in which psychological support is needed but cannot be easily incorporated in most health care systems.

Surgical Decisions and Patient Participation

Figure 1 indicates the possible outcomes that may follow biopsy and the reality to which the patient must adjust [28]. If a benign lesion is found, the incident is generally incorporated quickly, although anxiety is associated with knowledge of higher biologic vulnerability by virtue of genetic risk or fibrocystic disease. The recent increased attention to risk factors and early detection has in fact created a sense of heightened vulnerability for many women. The physician can be helpful by acknowledging and addressing the patient's fears. Reassurance about routine surveillance behaviors, including regular check-ups and instruction in breast self-examination, as well as awareness of physician availability should a symptom appear, all aid in the management of anxiety.

Breast cancer varies in its presentation and potential threat to life: treatment is determined by the location and stage of the tumor when detected [29]. The extent of the primary surgical procedure, and whether adjuvant therapy is necessary, poses major differences in the psychological stress of breast cancer. In recent years, women have become far better informed about the types of treatment and their meaning insofar as threat to life is concerned. They know more about lymph nodes involvement, for example, and that a recommendation for chemotherapy derives from the increased threat to life by possible micrometastasis from positive nodes. In addition, the side-effects

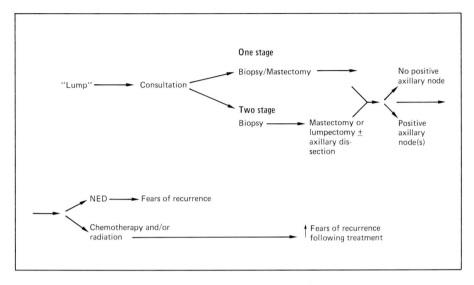

Fig. 1. The possible clinical courses following breast biopsy.

of the adjuvant therapies (chemotherapy and/or radiation) complicate adjustment and must be tolerated shortly after recovery from surgery itself.

The choice of primary surgical intervention is controversial and presents a new dilemma for those women who seek available information to participate in treatment decisions. Although the modified radical mastectomy has been the primary treatment of choice for primary breast cancer, conservative breast-saving surgery plus local irradiation has been increasingly advocated by some breast surgeons and radiotherapists as an acceptable alternative to mastectomy for the treatment of tumors under 3 cm [30].

Today, a total reversal has occurred in which women are given detailed survival statistics by treatment modality; they then are left to make the choice among the treatment options. Several states now require this presentation of treatment options. This requires confrontation by the women with the fact that no treatment offers 100% protection and data do not clearly yet indicate which treatment is safest.

Women now sometimes request psychiatric consultation due to the distress of having to make such a decision. Since segmental resection and radiation is new, many women fear that they may be compromising survival for appearance or 'vanity'. Even a well informed, educated decision is subject to fearful questioning during periods of post-treatment anxiety about recurrence.

Physician support can be instrumental in reducing self-doubt. This potential for self-doubt or guilt is clearly one of the 'new' psychological stresses that was not a problem when patients did not participate in the planning of treatment. The recent assumption of responsibility on the part of the patient is important, but it adds a new and an additional burden during an already stressful period.

When a patient chooses lumpectomy, she may or may not undergo axillary dissection to establish status of axillary nodes. She is generally advised then to undergo several weeks of radiation therapy. Treatments are done on an out-patient basis and begin about 4–6 weeks following surgery. Treatment side effects are moderately distressing but the patient feels that 'something is being done' and that she is under continuous surveillance. Anxiety may emerge when treatment is completed and she is on her own for the first time in many weeks or months without the 'protection of treatment' and the reassurance of weekly physician's visits [31].

When chemotherapy is required, the increased threat to life is recognized. Breast reconstruction must be often postponed and new problems must be faced. The side-effects of chemotherapy include fatigue, nausea and vomiting, hair loss and premature menopause which may or may not be reversible. The loss of vitality and childbearing potential, plus change in appearance, are sources of great emotional distress.

When a mastectomy is done, its impact relates to the point in the life cycle at which it occurs, and what social tasks are threatened or interrupted. The threat to femininity and self esteem occurs in *all* women, but it may be greater for a young woman whose attractiveness and fertility are paramount, or for those without a close sexual relationship. The patient's interpersonal environment is particularly significant in adaptation to the loss [29].

Rehabilitation and Reconstructive Surgery

The rehabilitation that is currently available is also extremely important in psychological adaptation. New protheses or breast forms, which have been developed with greater concern for matching shape, size and color, as well as specifically designed clothes, have made adjustment easier than in the past. Most important, reconstructive breast surgery has become increasingly available. Information about this option, which is now often presented prior to mastectomy, helps to diminish some of the profound sense of loss and finality previously associated with mastectomy.

Recent studies done by the psychiatric group at Memorial Sloan-Kettering have found that women seeking reconstructive surgery following mastectomy had realistic expectations about outcome, often pursued it for personal reasons, at times over family objections and had a high level of psychosocial functioning [32].

That breast reconstruction can improve the quality of life for many women has been demonstrated [33–35]. A number of researchers point out that the most often cited motives for this surgery are pragmatic issues of physical comfort and less restricted wardrobe. Expectations for change reflect the disequilibrium associated with mastectomy, rather that anticipation of a magical change in life circumstances related to breast cancer surgery [36, 37]. That satisfaction with outcome seems to be uniformly high also attests to the soundness of patients' expectations.

The psychological value of the procedure is most evident in the repetitive themes heard following reconstruction. Many women report feeling more physically comfortable and attractive, self-confident and relaxed, and with greatly improved morale. This change in self-evaluation is also apparent in a return to more satisfactory sexual relations, which are often impaired following mastectomy. Interestingly, there are suggestions that just the fact the option *exists* following mastectomy is reassuring in itself, even if it is not exercised [32, 38].

Although the stresses posed by the clinical course of diagnosis, treatment and rehabilitation are considerable, most patients are able to respond with only transient psychological distress which improves over time. A recent controlled prospective study by *Bloom* et al. followed up on women a year after mastectomy and compared them to a matched sample of women who had had a cholecystectomy, a negative breast biopsy or no current health problems. All groups were screened to *exclude* women with prior psychiatric disturbances [39]. Among those who had a mastectomy, moderate levels of psychological impairment were found which diminished over 12 months. However, the prevalence of severe psychiatric disturbances was *not* greater in the mastectomy group. These data are important in the current climate of breast-conserving surgery when decisions are sometimes made on the basis of anticipated psychological problems associated with mastectomy. That is, for most women severe psychological problems do not appear due to mastectomy in women who are psychologically healthy.

For some patients, however, adjustment is more difficult. Such women experience more that the usual level of distressing symptoms, sometimes to the point of serious psychological decompensation requiring intervention.

The ability to identify these women early remains a problem, but the presence of pre-existing psychological problems poses a significant risk factor.

Psychiatric Syndromes

The psychiatric syndromes outlined by *Holland and Mastrovito* in breast cancer are discussed below [29].

Perioperative Syndromes

The stress responses which occur just before the time of surgery are referred to as perioperative psychiatric syndromes. They are characterized by the presence of situational anxiety, depression or a mixture of both, particularly pre-operatively. Acutely, the patients may be unable to perform daily tasks, with insomnia, anorexia and weight loss. The response has phases characterized by denial, emotional distress, and resolution similar to phases which occur in acute grief. The response is apt to be characterized by a high level of anxiety. An important concern is that the level of anxiety may interfere with reasonable judgement about accepting proper medical care.

The key to the management of this pre-operative stress lies with the surgeon. In consultative visits, the surgeon should establish a relationship with the patient that conveys confidence in surgical ability using an approach which promotes a sense of trust and interest and which shows a willingness to discuss treatment options and answer questions.

Post-Operative Syndromes

The post-operative syndromes are of two kinds: stress responses and the more serious complication of post-operative delirium/psychosis occurring in the immediate post-operative period. (Post-operative delirium is more fully discussed on p. 51.) The most common problems are transient stress reactions to the loss of a meaningful body part and readaption to prior social and sexual roles. The radical mastectomy, done commonly until the last five years, produced more functional disability, greater disfigurement of the chest wall, and a more severe reaction, particularly when the surgery had to be kept a secret from others. Even today, however, with modified or less extensive removal of breast tissue, there is still a reaction to loss of a body part which has emotional meaning both in relation to attractiveness, sexuality and nurturing. The usual post-operative response is a form of normal grief. Women do better when they are prepared for the fact that they may have the 'blues', cry easily, and feel more anxious and depressed for a few weeks after the operation. Nightmares may be frightening and reflect unexpressed fears of bodily damage, death and fears of rejection by the sexual partner. It is at this time that the surgeon may need to be most supportive. Ancillary medical and paramedical forces are usually of great help, but the treating physician (surgeon) must be aware that he or she is the key figure from whom the patient needs support. Thus, the surgeon must be prepared to accept, in a supportive manner, the patient's distress and sometimes hostility.

Maladjustment During Rehabilitation

Most women return, over 1 to 3 months, to normal home life and work, with a gradual return to usual energy levels and normal spirit. *Penman* found that women who were at high risk of a continued level of distress at four months could be identified by their less effective coping strategies employed in the immediate post-operative period [40]. Anti-anxiety medication such as diazepam (Valium) 2–5 mg can diminish tension and encourage a more relaxed response to social situations. Evidence supports the fact that psychotropic medication used in such a setting is readily given up when the stressful time is over.

Psychosexual difficulties may arise as a stress response either in the patient or her sexual partner. As a response to both surgery and to the emotional stress temporarily manifested by having little sexual desire, the patient may suffer a threat to self-esteem. She may also fear being rejected and may transiently become frigid and distant as result of these feelings, at a time when the need for affection and sexual attention is actually heightened and strongly desired but also feared. The male partner, because of fears of inflicting injury or pain during intercourse, may also experience difficulties with sexual performance. The mastectomy may actually threaten the male's own sense of body integrity and invulnerability, making sexual relations difficult. The best treatment in these situations is *prevention* – by instructions from the surgeon. He/she should: outline how soon sexual relations may be resumed; indicate that intercourse will not result in injury; express the belief that resumption of usual sexual activity is an important aspect of rehabilitation. Moreover, the surgeon should express an interest in his/her patient's sexual concerns, and above all, listen for questions and encourage them.

Reactions to Adjuvant Therapy

Adjuvant therapy after mastectomy may be either radiotherapy or chemo-therapy; both are frightening since they represent evidence of a continuing threat to life and another threat to body integrity and function, just when adjustment to a mastectomy is being accomplished. The advice given by the radiotherapist or oncologist in initial consultation is critical in providing the patient with accurate information about the need for treatment, alternatives, side effects, risks and benefits. The physician's manner should convey a sense of confidence about the treatment plan by answering questions and establishing a therapeutic alliance.

Psychological preparation for treatment should include meeting the clinic nurse, staff, and particularly the nurse who will give the chemotherapy or the technician operating the radiotherapy machine. The psychological rehearsal allows anticipation of the treatment and significantly diminishes anxiety. (On p. 23 are discussed pre-treatment anxieties of surgical patients and their somewhat analogous management.) The attitudes and manner of the entire clinic staff, from the secretary who greets the patient each day to the technician and the physician, become positive adaptive forces in the patient's experience of the treatment setting.

Central Nervous System Complications

There are three common causes of central nervous system complications in breast cancer. In order of frequency, they are: metastatic brain lesions, metabolic encephalopathy and drug-induced encephalopathy [29]. The onset of altered behavior in a woman who has breast cancer, particularly if sudden, must be carefully assessed for possible cerebral dysfunction. A change in mood, apathy or loss of interest in surroundings, should also be cause for consideration, not only of functional causes but also for central nervous system complications of breast cancer. A brain metastasis may be the first indication of dissemination. As women receive more aggressive and effective primary treatment for breast cancer, more survive longer, increasing the likelihood of distant metastases, particularly intracerebral metastases which are increasing in frequency.

In the presence of known disseminated disease with bone metastases, hypercalcemia commonly produces a metabolic encephalopathy with a fluctuating picture of mild delirium, confusion, depressed mood, and intellectual deficit. (Delirium is further discussed on p. 51.)

The third area of central nervous system complications results from drugs. A number of different narcotics given for analgesia can produce idiosyncratic responses with hallucinations and acute delirium. Another drug that can produce striking mental symptoms are cortico-steroids. Steroids are a common part of adjuvant treatment and management of advanced disease. Although commonly causing mood changes, only infrequently do they produce psychosis.

Summary

Breast cancer has been the most carefully studied site of tumor from a psychological point of view. A range of interventions have been developed to assist the woman and her family in the emotional adjustment to breast cancer and its treatment. Many of these have been developed 'by women for women' and by their insistence that the medical community give more attention to this aspect of medical care. Rehabilitation now centers far more on breast reconstruction then previously. The psychologic understanding of problems posed by breast cancer has been used to develop rational and appropriate psychosocial interventions to reduce emotional distress. This model for development of support in breast cancer should be applied to psychologic management of patients with cancers of other sites, particularly those that carry high emotional distress and that place extensive demand on an individual's adaptive capacities.

References

1   Meyerowitz, B.E.: Psychosocial correlates of breast cancer and its treatment. Psychol. Bull. 8: 108–131 (1980).
2   Bard, M.; Sutherland, A.M.: Psychological impact of cancer and its treatment. IV. Adaptation to radical mastectomy. Cancer 8: 652–672 (1955),
3   Surveillance Epidemiology and End Results: Incidence and Mortality Data, 1973–1977,

Young, J.L.; Percy, C.L.; Asire, A. (eds.), National Cancer Institute Monograph, 57, N.I.H. Publication # 81-2330, U.S. Dept. of Health and Human Services.

4   Schottenfeld, D.; Robbins, G.F.: Quality of survival among patients who have had radical mastectomy. Cancer 26: 650–654 (1970).

5   Craig, T.J.; Comstock, G.W.; Geiser, P.B.: The quality of survival in breast cancer: a case-control comparison. Cancer 33: 1451–1457 (1974).

6   Maquire, G.P.; Lere, E.G.; Bevington, D.J.; Kuchermann, C.J.; Crabtree, R.J.; Cornell, C.E.: Psychiatric problems in the first year after mastectomy: a two year follow-up study. Brit. Med. J. 1: 163–165 (1978).

7   Lee, E.; Maguire, G.O.: Emotional distress of patients attending a breast clinic. Brit. J. Surg. 62: 162 (1975).

8   Crile, G.: Management of breast cancer: limited mastectomy. J. Am. Med. Ass. 230: 95–98 (1974).

9   Halstead, W.S.: The results of operations for care of cancer of the breast performed at John Hopkins Hospital from June, 1899 to January 1989. Ann. Surg. 20: 497–550 (1898).

10 Anglem, T.J.: Management of breast cancer; radical mastectomy. J. Am. Med. Ass. 230: 99–105 (1974).

11 Fisher, B.; Barboni, P.: Breast cancer chapter XXVIII, in Holland, J.F.; Frei, E. III, eds., Cancer Medicine, 2nd ed., pp. 2025–2056 (Lea & Febrler, Philadelphia 1982).

12 Veronesi, U.; Sacozzi, R.; Delvecchi, M.; et al.: Comparing radical mastectomy with quadrantectomy, axillary dissection and radiotherapy in patients with small cancer of the breast. N. Eng. J. Med. 205: 6–11 (1981).

13 Harris, J.B.; Levine, M.B.; Hellmann, S.: Results of treating stage I and II carcinoma of the breast with primary radiation therapy. Cancer Treat. Rep. 62: 985–991 (1978).

14 Rosato, F.; Horton, C.L.; Maxwell, G.O.: Post-mastectomy breast reconstruction. Curr. Probl. Surg. XVII: 11 (1980).

15 Watts, G.T.: Restorative prosthetic mammoplasty in mastectomy for carcinoma and benign lesions. Clin. Plast. Surg. 3: 177–191 (1976).

16 Mendelson, B.C.. The evolution of breast reconstruction. After 86 years, breast reconstruction has become a safe, simple and practical operation. Med. J. Aust. 1: 7 (1982).

17 Breslow, L.: Early case-finding, treatment and mortality from cervix and breast cancer. Prev. Med. 1: 141 (1972).

18 Dodd, G.W.: Present status of mammography, ultrasound and thermography in breast cancer detection. Paper presented at: Breast Cancer: A report to the Profession, sponsored by The White House: National Cancer Institute; America Cancer Society, (Washington, D.C., November 222–23 1976).

19 Hungerly, C.; Brown, R.: The value of breast self-examination. Cancer 47: 989–995 (1981).

20 Schwartz, G.: Risk factors in breast cancer: a clinical approach. Breast 8 (1): 26–29 (1982).

21 Schain, W.S.: Physician-patient responsibility in breast cancer management: the value of patient participation, in Schwartz, G.; Marchant, D., eds., Breast disease, diagnosis and treatment, pp. 251–274 (Elsevier-North Holland, Inc., Phil 1981).

22 Kushner, R.: Breast cancer: a personal history and investigative report. (Harcourt, Brace & Jovanovich, N.Y. 1975).

23 Antonovsky, A.; Hartman, H.: Delay in the detection of cancer: review of the literature. Health Educ. Monogr. 2: 98 (1974).

24 Howe, H.L.: Enhanced effectiveness of media, Publ. Health Repts. 96 (2): 134–142 (1981).

25   Beahrs, O.H.; Shapiro, S.; Smart, C.: Report of the working group to review the National Cancer Institute breast cancer demonstration projects. J. Nat. 1. Ca. Inst. *62:* 641–709 (1979).

26   Bernay, T.: The impact of breast cancer screening on feminine identity: Implications for patient education. Breast *8* (1): 2–5 (1982).

27   Katz, J.L.; Weinger, H.; Gallagher, T.F.; Hellman, L.: Stress, distress and ego defenses: psychoendocrine response to impending breast biopsy. Arch. Gen. Psych. *23:* 131–142 (1970).

28   Holland, J.: The clinical course of breast cancer: a psychological perspective. Front. Radiat. Ther. Onc. *11:* 33–145 (1976).

29   Holland, J.C.; Mastrovito, R.: Psychologic adaptation to breast cancer. Cancer *46:* 1045–1052 (1980).

30   Consumer Reports, Breast Cancer: the retreat from radical surgery, January 24–30 (1981).

31   Holland, J.C.; Rowland, J.; Lebovits, A.; Rusalem, R.: Reactions to cancer treatments: Assessment of emotional reactions to adjuvant radiotherapy as a guide to planned intervention. Psych. Clin. N. A. *2:* 347–358 (1979).

32   Jacobs, E.; Holland, J.; et al.: Reconstructive breast surgery after mastectomy: A comparative study of psychological aspects. Proc. XIII International Cancer Congress, p. 24, Abstract # 938–167, 1982.

33   Rowland, J.; Holland, J.C.: Breast reconstruction: Issues in management and support. Annual Meeting, Society of Behavioral Medicine (Philadelphia, May 1984).

34   Rowland, J.; Holland, J.C.; Jacobs, E.R.; Chaglassiant, T.; Geller, N.; Petroni, G.; Kovachev, D.; Kinne, D.: Psychological responses to breast reconstruction. Annual APA Meeting (Los Angeles ca. 1984).

35   Zalon, J.; Block, J.L.: I am whole again. (Random House, New York 1978).

36   Schain, W.S.: Psychosocial Issues in Counseling Mastectomy Patients. Couns. Psychol. *6:* 45–49 (1976).

37   Goin, J.M.; Goin, M.K.: Changing the body: Psychological effects of plastic surgery (Williams & Wilkins Co., Baltimore, Md. 1981).

38   Schain, W.S.; Jacobs, E.R.; Wellisch, D.K.: Psychosocial issues in breast reconstruction: intrapsychic, interpersonal and practical concerns. Clin. Plast. Surg. *11:* 237–251 (1984).

39   Bloom, J.; Cook, M.; Holland, J.; Muenz, L.: A prospective comparison study of women's psychological response to mastectomy. Psychological adjustment to breast cancer cooperative group, NCI, ASCO Abstracts # C-284:273 (1984).

40   Penman, D.: Coping with mastectomy. Doctoral dissertation, Yeshiva University (1979).

J. Holland, MD, Cornell University Medical College and Chief, Psychiatry Service, Memorial Sloan-Kettering Cancer Center, New York, NY 10021 (USA)

Adv. psychosom. Med., vol. 15, pp. 124–139 (Karger, Basel 1986)

Psychiatric Aspects of Cardiac Surgery

Stanley Heller[a], Donald Kornfeld[b]

[a] Associate Clinical Professor of Psychiatry College of Physicians and Surgeons at Columbia University and Director, C/L Services St. Luke Roosevelt Hospital, New York, N.Y., USA
[b] Columbia University, College of Physicians and Surgeons, and Chief, Consultation Liaison Psychiatry Service Presbyterian Hospital, New York, N.Y., USA

Each of the three decades of cardiac surgery has had a dominant focus. Initially it was closed mitral commissurotomy, later followed by open heart surgery, primarily of valvular and congenital defects, and most recently coronary artery bypass grafting (CABG). The next decade will probably witness the further development of artificial hearts and progress in transplantation.

Early on, cardiac surgery, with the high incidence of post-cardiotomy delirium, was a virtual laboratory of delirium research. Surgery in the 1960's, on large numbers of chronic heart patients with valvular disease, also led to problems in adaptation, as persons with life-long illness had to cope with new-found health.

In this chapter, we will review psychological and psychiatric factors sequentially through the cardiac surgery process, i.e., pre-operative, operative and post-operative phases. We will examine outcome studies of open heart and CABG surgery. Finally, we will consider heart transplantation and the prospect of the availability of an artificial heart as it raises additional questions regarding man's adaptation to technology.

Pre-Operative Considerations

While the specific cardiac operations may have changed, an understanding of patients' personality profiles and motivations for surgery continues to have relevance as predictors of clinical outcome. In one of the earliest such studies, *Kennedy and Bakst* [1] found a variety of attitudes in patients seeking surgery. Some patients were illness deniers, others were disease dependent, some terrified of surgery. Intermediate, conflicted positions also existed with some seeking freedom from illness while simultaneously fearing to give up their dependent roles. A small group of suicidal patients were found hoping for surgical death. Others had psychiatric illness masquerading as cardiac illness. This last group is now less likely to come to surgery since cardiac diagnostic measures are so much more precise.

Using a similar classification system, *Kimball* [2] placed patients preoperatively into four categories in an effort to predict operative and post-operative course. 'Adjusted' patients were psychologically healthy and realistic. 'Symbiotic' patients were illness-dependent. 'Anxious' patients, although denying anxiety, showed it in their behavior. 'Depressed' patients had 'given in' and then 'given up' and were poorly motivated for surgery. The 'adjusted' patients did best 15 months later with ¾ having a benign recovery. On the other hand, 'symbiotic' patients had prolonged convalescence and a poor outcome with only 7% rated improved. 'Anxious' patients had a 25% surgical mortality, often with arrythmias and variable outcome. Depressed patients fared the worst with a 79% death rate and a poor outcome for the survivors.

Another conflicted group has been identified by *Blacher and Cleveland* as suffering from survivor guilt [3]. These patients wonder if they deserve relief from an illness that killed a parent. The authors suggest that pre-operative psychotherapeutic intervention may be needed to avoid post-operative depression. Post-operative therapy for the depressed patient required an interpretation of the underlying guilt-provoking mechanism. It was acknowledged for the patient that pleasure over the prospect of cure is difficult as one remembers the deaths of family members from similar problems. Relief was also facilitated by pointing out to the patient that the operation had not been available to an earlier generation.

Throughout the history of cardiac surgery, psychiatrists have been asked to evaluate patients who refuse needed surgery or are made massively anxious by it. While minor tranquilizers may be helpful in dealing with the overly anxious patient, some may need a 'phobic companion' who will give them the equivalent of a safe conduct pass through the operation. Some patients will need behavior therapy and desensitization to the hospital and operating room setting; however, care must be taken not to elicit too much anxiety in patients with advanced cardiac disease.

Patients may also decline surgery because they are severely depressed. In effect the patient is saying: 'Life is so painful and with so few pleasures, why should I bother to go through something as difficult as cardiac surgery?' If the surgery is elective, it should be postponed until after the treatment of the depression. A severely depressed person is at heightened risk post-operatively because of poor cooperation and compliance in the immediate post-operative period. The physiological changes associated with severe major depression can probably also contribute to the increased morbidity and mortality in these patients.

Some obsessive-compulsive patients may be admitted to the hospital and cancel their surgery only hours beforehand. Such patients may be motivated by an unconscious need to remain in control. The passivity of the general anesthesia and surgical patient role over-ride all realistic considerations of health.

Just as excessive anxiety may lead to problems, the denial of anxiety may also lead to post-operative difficulties. Patients who have not experienced and expressed their pre-operative anxiety may react in a hostile, paranoid way following the pain and scarring of surgery [4, 5]. Moreover, they have not been able to reach out for support from families and staff due to their need to appear tough and independent. Such patients benefit considerly from psychiatric consultation that encourages ventilation [6]. The extent of pre-operative denial is illustrated by the study of *Thurer* et al. [7] who reported on common patient misperceptions of their impending cardiac surgery. Many patients misstated the operative mortality statistics as a one in 10,000 chance of death or 'not a (bad) chance in a million', others misperceived the nature of the operation itself: e.g., $\frac{1}{4}$ of coronary artery bypass patients thought the heart was removed from the body during the surgery, and another $\frac{1}{4}$ were not sure, while 10% thought the heart was cut open during the procedure. The authors found that patients often displaced their anxiety on to incidental issues such as needles or troublesome roommates. Recent nightmares were also common. Idealization of the surgeon as 'God', 'Golden Hands', 'the best in the business' was common especially among deniers of anxiety.

A majority of the coronary artery bypass surgery group patients manifest the coronary prone behavior pattern (type A). These patients are less likely to express anxiety and therefore, have less available social support. These individuals have difficulty in assuming the dependent role, and therefore may have particular problems in the open-heart recovery room. One study found that the very independent type was more likely to suffer from post-cardiotomy delirium [5]. Care is facilitated if these reactions are anticipated, the staff acknowledging that the patient is an independent person who will have difficulties in the dependent role. The staff should be alerted and told to take a more active role in providing support, even if it is not requested. The independent patient should be told that the assumption of the totally dependent role will take great fortitude. This very accurate observation often allows such a patient to better tolerate the distress imposed by dependency.

Blacher [8] has explored the inner world of the patient awaiting cardiac surgery and has elucidated fantasies of death and rebirth. Patients struggle with the concept of their hearts not beating during surgery – shouldn't that mean they are dead, if only for a while? Religious patients may anticipate that dead relatives may be rejoined during this time. Exposure of these fantasies can lead to resolution of pre-operative anxiety. *Blacher* also suggested that the observation made by some patients that their mortality risk was '50%' (rather than 1%) may be due to the patient's perception of a heart which either beats or stops. (For further discussion of pre-operative reactions, refer to p. 1, Pre-operative emotional states and post-operative recovery and p. 23, Psychological intervention with surgical patients: evaluation outcome.)

Post-Cardiac Surgery Delirium

The major immediate post-operative problem remains post-cardiotomy delirium, a cognitive impairment often with accompanying perceptual aberrations. The syndrome was first described in 1964 [9–11], and typically develops several days post-operatively after a lucid interval. It may begin with illusions triggered by sounds in the open heart recovery room and progress to hallucinations and paranoid delusions. Up to 70% of patients [11] were afflicted in early studies; however, the incidence has declined in recent years to approximately 25% [12]. The more recent reports reflecting current trends in cardiac surgery are primarily for patients undergoing CABG [12–15]. Research in post-operative psychiatric problems has been confused by some investigators who have failed to distinguish between the various forms of psychopathology which can occur. For example, delirium may occur immediately upon awakening from anesthesia (the early organic brain syndrome) or after a lucid interval of two to four days. The etiological elements are quite different in these two phenomena. Some studies have also included affective disorders, an obviously very different problem. Further research into etiological factors may be aided by a proposed international study using standardized nomenclature, instruments, samples and data gathering procedures [16].

In their first study, the *Columbia group* suggested that a combination of pre-operative, operative and post-operative factors play a role in delirium [11]. Research by many groups over the past 20 years has confirmed this hypothesis and demonstrated the complexity of multiple factors at work. The early reports noted such factors as age, severity and length of illness; intra-operatively, length of operative time, pump time, and hypotension [17]; and post-operatively length of time in the Open Heart Recovery Room (OHRR) with its associated sensory, motor and sleep deprivation [17–20]. It has been shown (21, 22) that cardiac surgery has been associated with persistent sleep disturbances and EEG abnormalities that last 2 to 4 weeks post-operatively. No REM sleep is probable until the fourth post-operative night.

While reduction in pump time has been associated with decreased incidence in delirium [18], no one factor may account for the reduced incidence. Among the myriad of contributing factors associated with the pump alone are: stabilizing agents, particulate matter from extracorporeal circuit, silicone emboli, protein denaturation, cavitation bubbles, pebbles and particles from the priming fluids, low oxygenator levels, excessive hemodilution, low cerebral blood flow, high brain venous pressure and microbubble emboli [23]. In one study, routine EEG monitoring during bypass discovered 5 patients that had unsuspected poor cerebral blood flow, thereby alerting pump technicians for the need to correct a mechanical problem [24].

In a more recent study, post-operative cardiac output has also been implicated. Increased delirium was found in mitral valve repair patients whose generally low cardiac output failed to increase, or patients with aortic valve replacements whose cardiac outputs decreased [25].

The *Columbia group* [3] found that pre- and post-operative ventilation contributed to delirium prevention. Patients who had a continuous relationship with the research team both before and after surgery had a 50% reduction in delirium incidence compared to a non-followed sample. It was felt that research interviews served a prophylactic and therapeutic function by creating a reassuring atmosphere and implicit alliance during this stressful time [3, 25]. Patients with an active dominant personality were found to be more likely to develop delirium, presumably because these persons were unable to acknowledge their anxiety or assume a dependent role. This attitude deprived them of the opportunity for emotional support.

Layne and Yudofsky [6] found that lower pre-operative anxiety scores, based on self-report, were associated with a higher incidence of delirium. They recommended that special efforts be made to get such denying patients to express their emotions about the operation prior to surgery.

It was also found that patients who received more tranquilizers had a higher rate of delirium [5]. Tranquilized patients were also physically sicker and more vulnerable on that basis. No significant interaction was found between anxiety level and tranquilizer use.

Delirium after coronary artery bypass graft surgery (CABG) is not literally 'post cardiotomy' since the heart is not extensively opened. Moreover, during CABG the heart is beating and being perfused, causing less cardiac damage and making air embolization less likely. Delirium rates reported following CABG are in the 25% range. Many of the previously associated variables, such as severity of illness, length of bypass time and age failed to correlate with delirium. Severity of recovery room illness has remained a risk factor, and a new risk factor for delirium has been uncovered: history of myocardial infarction. Previous infarction may have been associated with a previous history of cerebral anoxia or may have contributed to diminished cardiac output post-operatively, making the patients more vulnerable. Although active dominant personalities were not at higher risk, a related finding was that confidence and composure were suggestively correlated with delirium [12].

The complexity of the post-cardiotomy delirium problem is revealed by the following list of correlates of post surgical delirium in a single study [19]: abnormal EEG, albuminuria, anemia, azotemia, hypochloremia, hypokalemia, hyponatremia, cardiac failure, cardio-vascular disease, infection, intoxication, more than 5 drugs pre-operatively, procedure lasting more than 4 hours, emergency operation, post-operative complications and more than 5 drugs post-operation.

Treatment

How can one best prevent or treat post-cardiotomy delirium? A pre-operative visit from the nursing staff can help develop a trusting relationship. Patients should be told pre-operatively that a delirium may occur. They should be encouraged to communicate all such symptoms to the staff. They should be reassured that, should this occur, it is a common and temporary problem. Patients who are unprepared may fear that they are 'going crazy' or that they have suffered permanent brain damage. Patients should be transferred from the Open Heart Recovery Room to a more normal hospital environment as soon as feasible. While in the OHRR every effort should be made to reduce sleep interruption and increase the patient's mobility. Family visiting should be encouraged and translators provided to non-English speaking patients. The staff should provide orientation cueing.

Should the delirium develop, every effort should be made to find a specific etiology, e.g., drug effects, metabolic abnormalities, etc. Should these not be present, one can assume that some noxious element in the environment has triggered or produced a post-cardiotomy delirium. For most patients transfer out of the OHRR can produce an improvement in 24–48 hours. Where that is not possible or transfer alone does not produce improvement, anti-psychotic medication is indicated. A more sedating phenothiazine to help provide sleep, such as chlorpromazine can be used, provided small doses are used (12.5–25 mg i.m.) and the patient's blood pressure is monitored. (For further discussion of post-operative delirium, refer to p. 51.)

Following surgery, patients should have the opportunity to review and understand their psychotic experiences and fears. Again they should be reassured that this is a common occurrence and in no way reflects on their emotional stability.

Later post-operative reactions, particularly depression, have not been studied as extensively. Survivor guilt [3] may be a contributing factor. Unexpressed hostility to doctors may also play a role particularly if there are complications such as wound infection. Half the patients identify the endotracheal tube as the worst aspect of their surgery. Nursing care is often the subject of complaints although many patients spontaneously praise a staff member, often of the same ethnicity.

Generally surgeons continue to be praised with anger displaced onto the hospital, calling it 'impersonal, a dungeon', even 'a slaughterhouse'. Anger and depression may also be triggered by an uncertainty of the prognosis.

Transient post-operative depression may occur as a form of psychological and physiological 'let down' following the great stress of the pre-operative period. Whether patients having the surgery on an elective basis with a relatively long pre-operative period of stress are more prone to depression than patients who undergo an emergency procedure is an open question.

Post-operative assessment of intellectual functioning has shown that most patients do not suffer any significant decrement of function. An improvement in pre- to post-scores has been found and patients who had been delirious did no worse than average [26]. When carefully screened post-operatively, about 10% of patients are found to show an impairment that improves, in the areas of visuo-spatial relations, perception, and cognition. Long perfusion times, valvular calcification and intra-operative complications correlate with poorer performance [27–29]. The insertion of a micropore filter was found to decrease cognitive impairment [29] suggesting an etiologic role for micro-emboli. When seen very soon after surgery, more patients will show EEG and neuro-psychological abnormalities, particularly if compromised pre-operatively [29]. It has been recently reported [30] that leakage of adenylate kinase from brain cells correlates with intellectual impairment post-operatively.

In general, operative mortality rates correlate with extent of central nervous system dysfunction. Indeed neuropsychological testing can be a quality criterion for surgery [29].

The repair of valvular and congenital defects provided patients with the prospect of longer, more productive lives. For some, however, there was psychological decline in the face of this physical improvement.

Outcome Studies

Valvular Surgery

The earliest follow up of psychological functioning was done by the *Blachlys* in 1968 [31]. Despite near universal benefit, 40% of their patients were unable to hold a job or do housework. In a finding later repeated many times, they discovered that prolonged unemployment (greater than one year) made return to work unlikely. A later study by *Lucia and McGuire* [32] of valve surgery patients was more favorable, with improved functioning in all areas. 3/4 of their patients were doing 'more', while only 1/6 were doing less than pre-operatively. The *Columbia group* [33] studied almost 1,000 members of the Mended Hearts Society, a self-help organization of former cardiac surgical patients. 90% were pleased to have had the operation, but 1/6 acknowledged that psychological factors may have impeded their recovery. Sexual function was the least improved area and there were complaints of overprotective families and inadequate and insufficiently detailed physician advice.

In a 1970 study, the *Columbia group* [34] found 1/3 of open heart surgery patients described a general decline in adjustment despite physical improvement. There was a tendency to passivity and impaired sexual and marital functioning. A high risk pre-operative group was identified as those patients who were disorganized, highly anxious and with a paranoid tendency. At the other extreme, aggressive unreflective patients also had problems as they were unable to submit to dependent care. Pre-operative depression and reluctance to agree to surgery also correlated with poor outcome.

Coronary Artery Bypass Surgery

110,000 CABG procedures were performed in 1981, consuming 1% of total health care expenses [35]. There is considerable concern regarding the annual cost of over 2,000,000,000 dollars for this operation. In addition to survival, the quality of life issue is, therefore, being examined in detail. It became quickly apparent that there was insufficient improvement in employment rates to justify the surgery. However, *Weinstein* et al. [36] have shown that there was increased life span for patients with disease of the left anterior descending artery and with triple vessel disease.

Previous psychiatric and psychological research on valvular and congenital repair surgery has only limited relevance in the CABG population. CABG patients have generally not been burdened by long-standing congestive heart failure, and their frequently type A behavior stands in contrast to the passivity of the chronically ill cardiac patient. As with the cardiotomy operations, almost all CABG patients studied [37] were pleased they had undergone the operation. Only 4% regretted it, 3–4 years later. Over half the patients had become totally pain free (angina had been the usual indication for operation). $\frac{3}{4}$ of the patients had worked before the operation and $\frac{3}{4}$ were working 9 months after it. Failure to return to work correlated with severity of cardiac disease. Patients who returned to work were younger, had more improvement in angina and were more likely to be type A both before and after operation. Among those who were working 3–4 years later, $\frac{2}{3}$ felt increased satisfaction in their work. At that same interval, overall pleasure in life had improved substantially with improvements in mood, family and sexual satisfaction. Only 4% reported worsening in family relations while 23% found reduced sexual satisfaction.

A comparison of sexual frequency pre-operatively and at 9 months post-operatively revealed that before surgery 67% were sexually active at least once a week and 11% had no activity, while post-operatively only 38% were active once a week or more and 31% had no sexual activity.

At follow-up there was general compliance with physician instructions concerning smoking, weight gain, exercise and medication. There was comparatively little change in overall type A behavior. 9 months post-operatively, 75% were unchanged in type A rating, 7% were more type A and 18% less so. At 3–4 years, 31% thought they had slowed down greatly, 31% somewhat, 25% a little, 16% not at all and 7% pushed themselves harder. There was a substantial decline in job commitment, however, among extreme type A men. Severe post-operative angina correlated with reduction of type A behavior while physical improvement permitted resumption of full activity. It is not yet known if persistent type A behavior correlates with heightened mortality [38–40].

Less favorable results were obtained in a study of a largely blue collar, predominantly white, male population in rural North Carolina [41]. There patients had good physiological outcomes as measured by treadmill testing. However 1–2 years post surgery, 83% were unemployed and 57% sexually impaired. Patients with pre-operative symptoms of greater than eight months duration did particularly poorly. It was suggested that this reflected a damaged self-concept exacerbated by surgery. These farm and factory workers, salesmen and managers had constricted social lives, low self-esteem, lack of pleasure from close relationships and depression with distorted body image. The authors concluded that their patients' strenuous jobs, plus the impact of the surgery, given their limited education and income, interfered with recovery. Patients with type A behavior pattern were more likely to return to work but were not better adapted than type B's. The *North Carolina group* therefore, recommended limiting the period of unemployment prior to surgery.

A more optimistic outcome was described by *Jenkins* et al. [42] in a study of post-bypass patients using a subjective self-report approach. They found impressive improvements in many areas associated with quality of life. Anxiety, depression, fatigue and sleep problems diminished whole vigor and well being scores increased. Of 60 outcome measures, not one showed serious worsening, leading the authors to conclude that patients had returned to normal economic and social functioning.

Zyzanski et al. [43] utilized the Mended Hearts Society to gather data on a large population. Interestingly, they found that the number of operated arteries did not affect return to work, which was generally excellent for males. The returners had higher incomes and white collar jobs. Although the non-returners tended to be sicker, only a small minority had serious complications. Perhaps more importantly, non-returners had been sicker pre-operatively and for a longer interval. All men and women forced to retire had greater problems, suggesting that they were an appropriate group for counseling.

The repeated findings of correlation of return to work with recent employment and an above-poverty socio-economic level was confirmed by *Boulay* et al. [44]. Factors favoring return to work were: light work, greater educational level, younger age, shorter duration of illness, less angina, and no non-cardio-vascular illness. Rehabilitation was again suggested for those with a negative risk profile.

In another Montreal study [45], only 13% never returned to work. Some patients who did not return to work attributed that decision to physician's advice, while others indicated employer reluctance. It is unclear specifically what these patients were told; however, the operated patients' heightened sense of vulnerability may interact with some physicians' medical-legal timidity to encourage unnecessary invalidism.

Another intensive study of return to work was conducted among over 1,400 patients operated upon in Maine [46]. All retired and unemployed persons remained so post-operatively. Of those employed, only 17% retired at a mean age of 63. Among those disabled prior to survey, 45% had become employable and 41% found jobs post-operatively. Of those that were disabled, $\frac{1}{4}$ had psychiatric problems. Half of the disabled group were either asymptomatic or much improved. These authors also concluded that improved working rates justified the operation's expense.

It is essential in evaluating post-operative return to work that we distinguish between patients unable to return to work for physical reasons, those afraid to return, those kept from working by employer attitudes and those who choose to retire or accept a disability pension. Therefore, return to work cannot be used as a sole criterion for successful procedure. Many patients have particularly positive responses [7]. Some describe their happy, pain free outcome as part of a divine plan. They report that they appreciate their families more, have a lessened but appropriate, involvement in work, and a greater awareness of life. 'I love life more. I discover things that I never knew before – grass, trees, flowers, snow.'

Based on these research findings, the psychiatrist working with CABG patients should be concerned about excessive invalidism, sexual avoidance, passivity and depression. Patients should be particularly encouraged to ask their physicians when they can resume sexual activity. Physicians should also be encouraged to provide their patients with specific information. In addition, some patients will have to be helped to understand that they have moved from the acute to the recovery phase. The operation should be conceived of as restorative, rather than as an additional narcissistic injury. Overprotective families may also require psychotherapy, or some psychologically oriented counseling.

It makes no sense to bypass a blocked artery without addressing the associated behavioral factors. Almost all risk factors for coronary artery disease have a behavioral component: smoking, overeating, non-compliance with diet and medication, inadequate exercise and the type A behavior pattern. Excessive arousal with heightened sympathetic tone may well be present. In addition, delay in seeking care is often due to denial of cardiac symptoms, which is also modifiable. Treatment groups for type A patients are becoming more available. Relaxation training or biofeedback may also reduce harmful catecholamine surges.

Psychotherapy should focus on: reduction of excessive hostility, the need to derive pleasure from more than work, the importance of recreation and relaxation, and non-competitive and non-perfectionistic attitudes within families. The operation should be viewed as an opportunity to re-think life's priorities and meaning.

Cardiac Transplantation

Nowhere, of course, does the heart's symbolic meaning have more impact than in cardiac transplantation. The heart is seen as the center of love and loyalty – 'My heart is breaking' or 'My heart isn't in it'. Both donor families and recipient view cardiac transplantation with awe. There are not many psychiatric studies of individuals involved in this complex process since so few centers have active programs. However, it is worth summarizing what work has been done.

Studies of donors, usually accident victims, reveal that they come from families with both a history of heart disease and medical sophistication [47]. The deceased had expressed a wish for such a use, and the families wished to give meaning to the donor's death. Interest of the donor family in the recipient declined after 4–6 weeks, paralleling their own grief response. Secondary, or renewed grieving, was not seen if the recipient died.

Christopherson and Lunde [48] felt that only mental retardation or active psychosis in a recipient are contraindications to cardiac transplantation, as these conditions preclude cooperation and truly informed consent. Since many potential transplant recipients have had severe chronic cardiac disease, cerebral impairment may be present, rendering the evaluation of ultimate post-operative cerebral functioning and mental status difficult. According to their work, factors predictive of good post-operative adaptation include: family support for the patient to have the transplant, ability to discuss the possibility of death and a specific plan of how to best make use of the extended life-time which the procedure might provide.

What should the relationship be between the donor family and the recipient? *Kraft* found that the family of the recipient often felt that a relationship with the donor's family was an emotional drain [49]. The recipient family members often felt forced to share the grief of the donor family for their lost member. In turn, the donor's family felt the need to emphasize the noble humanitarian gesture and symbolism of the heart and the need to think of their loved one living on symbolically in the recipient. Hence the recipient family can become more comfortable thinking of the heart merely as a pump. The *Stanford group*, therefore, felt that personal contact between the donor and the recipient family would not be productive, except for very specific situations where there was a mutual desire for one such meeting.

Christopherson and Lunde found that most patients post-operatively showed only limited personality changes, and those changes were primarily accentuations of characteristics present before the transplantation. The use of steroids post-operatively can produce, however, all the usual psychiatric problems associated with these drugs, especially emotional lability, difficulties in concentration and heightened irritability [47, 48]. *Kraft* noted the marked improvement in mood associated with post-operative relief of symptoms [49].

A variety of psychodynamic mechanisms were called upon in the post-operative period. Both *Christopherson and Lunde* [47, 48] and *Kraft* [49] commented on the use of denial e.g., when patients became aware of the death of another transplant patient. *Kraft* reports that some male patients associated the receipt of a heart from a young male donor with increased virility; others expressed concern about receiving a heart from a female donor. For a majority of patients, the most important task became the need to compromise their high expectations with the emotional and physical burdens of post-transplant existence. (For further discussion of transplantation, refer to p. 167.)

The recent introduction of the artificial heart, even one with a cumbersome external pump, did not generate any apparent intrinsic problems. The recipient's problems were similar to of other cardiac surgery patients, with a form of post-cardiotomy delirium proving to be a recurrent troublesome problem.

Shortly before the first artificial heart recipient died, he too expressed the belief it had been worthwhile, and after his death his family understandably emphasized his contribution to science. Of course, he had been carefully chosen, and had an unusually close and supportive family. It is to be expected that even more than for coronary bypass surgery, the future debate will focus on the economic and ethical factors involved in the procedure. The financial cost will be considerable. Who should bear it? With a limited supply of hearts and/or financial resources, who shall be chosen as future recipients? Psychiatrists will be asked to participate in these discussions, as we were in the early days of renal dialysis. In fact, the first recipient of an artificial heart was chosen by a committee consisting of the surgeon, a cardiologist, a psychiatrist, a social worker and a nurse with any member having veto power. The psychiatric examination was aimed at uncovering disqualifying major psychiatric illness as well as identifying useful coping qualities such as motivation, adaptability, capacity to utilize support systems and ego maturity [50].

References

1   Kennedy, J.A.; Bakst, H.: The influences of emotions on the outcome of cardiac surgery. A predictive study, Bull. N.Y. Acad. Med. *42:* 811–849 (1966).

2   Kimball, C.P.: Psychological responses to the experience of open heart surgery – I. Am. J. Psychiat. *126:* 348–359 (1969).

3   Blacher, R.S.; Cleveland, R.J.: Paradoxical depression after heart surgery – I; in Speidel, H.; Rodewald, G. eds., Psychic and neurological dysfunctions after open heart surgery, pp. 141–143 (George Thieme Verlag; Stuttgard, New York 1980).

4   Janis, I.L.: Psychological stress (John Wiley and Sons, 1959).

5   Kornfeld, D.S.; Heller, S.S.; Frank, K.A.; et al.: Personality and psychological factors in postcardiotomy delirium. Arch. Gen. Psych. *31:* 249–253 (1974).

6   Layne, O.Z.; Yudofsky, S.C.: Post-operative psychosis in cardiotomy. The role of organic and psychiatric factors. New Eng. J. Med. *284:* 518–520 (1971).

7   Thurer, S.; Levine, F.; Thurer, R.: The psychodynamic impact of coronary bypass surgery. Int. J. Psychiat. Med. *10:* 273–290 (1980–81).

8   Blacher, R.: Death, ressurection and rebirth: Observation in cardiac surgery. Psychoanal. Quart. *52:* 56–72 (1983).

9   Blachly, P.H.; Starr, A.: Post-cardiotomy delirium. Am. J. Psychiat. *121:* 371–379 (1964).

10 Egerton, N.; Kay, J.H.: Psychological disturbances associated with open heart surgery. Brit. J. Psychiat. *110:* 433–439 (1964).

11 Kornfeld, D.S.; Zimberg, S.; Malm, J.R.: Psychiatric complications of open-heart surgery. New Eng. J. Med. *273:* 287–292 (1965).

12 Kornfeld, D.S.; Heller, S.S.; Frank, K.A.; et al.: Delirium after artery bypass surgery. J. Thorac. Cardiovasc. Surg. *76:* 93–96 (1978).

13 Rabiner, C.J.; Willner, A.E.; Fishman, J.: Psychiatric complications following coronary bypass surgery. J. Nerv. Ment. Disord. *160:* 324–347 (1975).

14 Willner, A.E.; Rabiner, C.F.; Wisoff, B.G.; et al.: Analogical reasoning and postoperative outcome. Arch. Gen. Psych. *33:* 255–259 (1976).

15 Sveinsson, I.S.: Postoperative psychosis after heart surgery. J. Thoracic Cardiovasc. Surg. *70:* 717–726 (1975).

16 Katz, J.M.: The International Study, presentation Second International Symposium on

Psychopathological and Neurological Dysfunctions Following Open Heart Surgery. (Milwaukee, WS, March 7, 1980).

17 Tufo, H.M.; Ostfeed, A.M.; Sjele, E.R.: Central nervous system dysfunction following open heart surgery. J. Am. Med. Ass. *212:* 1333–1340 (1970).

18 Heller, S.S.; Frank, K.A.; Malm, J.R.; et al.: Psychiatric complications of open heart surgery, a re-examination. New Eng. J. Med. *283:* 1015–1020 (1970).

19 Morse, R.M.: The relationship between psychopathology (delirium- and somatic-organic-pharmacologic) factors following open heart surgery; in Speidel, H.; Rodenwald, G., eds., Psychic and neurological dysfunctions after open-heart surgery, pp. 111–117 (Georg Thieme Verlag, Stuttgart, New York 1980).

20 Lipowski, Z.J.: Delirium, clouding of consciousness and confusion. J. Nerv. Ment. Dis. *145:* 227–255 (1967).

21 Orr, W.C.; Stahl, M.L.: Sleep disturbances after open heart surgery. Am. J. Cardiol. *39:* 196–201 (1977).

22 Elwell, E.L.; Francel, B.L.; Snyder, F.: A Polygraphic sleep study of five cardiotomy patients. Presentation, Annual meeting of the Association for the Psychophysiological Study of Sleep. (Jackson Hole, Wyoming 1974).

23 Longmore, D.: Causes of cerebral complications after open-heart surgery, in Speidel, H.; Rodenwald, G., eds., Psychic and neurological dysfunctions after open-heart surgery, pp. 76–91 (Georg Thieme Verlag, Stuttgart, New York 1980).

24 Salerno, T.A.; Lince, D.P.; White, D.N.; et al.: Monitoring of electroencephalogram during open heart surgery. J. Thorac. Cardiovasc. Surg. *76:* 97–100 (1978).

25 Heller, S.S.; Kornfeld, D.S.; Frank, K.A.; et al.: Postcardiotomy delirium and cardiac output. Am. J. Psychiat. *136:* 337–339 (1979).

26 Frank, K.A.; Heller, S.S.; et al.: Long-term effects of open-heart surgery on intellectual functioning. J. Thorac. Cardiovasc. Surg. *64:* 811–815 (1972).

27 Lazarus, H.; Hagens, S.H.: Prevention of psychosis following open heart surgery. Am. J. Psychiat. *124:* 1190–1195 (1968).

28 Staneml, K.A.; Juolasmaa, A.; Hokkanen, E.T.. Neuropsychologic outcome after open-heart surgery. Arch. Neurol. *38:* 2–8 (1981).

29 Aberg, T.; Kihlgreen, M.: Effect of open heart surgery in intellectual function. Scand. J. Thorac. Cardiovasc. Surg. Supp. *15:* 1–63 (1974).

30 Aberg, T.: Ischemic brain damage and open heart surgery. Lancet *1:* 113–141 (1982).

31 Blachly, P.H.; Blachly, B.J.: Vocational and emotional status of 263 patients after heart surgery. Circ. *38:* 524–533 (1968).

32 Lucia, W.; McGuire, L.B.: Rehabilitation and functional status after surgery for valvular heart disease. Arch. Int. Med. *126:* 995–1000 (1970).

33 Frank, K.A.; Heller, S.S.; Kornfeld, D.S.: A survey of adjustment to cardiac surgery. Arch. Int. Med. *130:* 735–738 (1972).

34 Heller, S.S.; Frank, K.A.; Kornfeld, D.S.; et al.: Psychological outcome following open heart surgery. Arch. Int. Med. *134:* 908–914 (1974).

35 Cohen, H.A.; Solnice, N.; Stephenson, A.: The financing of coronary artery bypass surg. Circ. *66,* Supp. III: 49–55 (1982).

36 Weinstein, M.C.; Sterson, W.B.: Cost effectiveness of coronary artery bypass surg. Circ. *66,* Supp. III: 56–66 (1982).

37 Kornfeld, D.S.; Heller, S.S.; Frank, K.A.; et al.: Psychological and behavioral responses after coronary artery bypass surgery. Circ. *66,* Supp. III: 24–28 (1982).

38 Friedman, M.; Thoreson, C.E.; Gill, J.J.; et al.: Feasibility of altering type A behavior patterns after myocardial infarction. Circ. 6: 83–92 (1982).

39 Ibrahim, M.A.; Feldman, J.G.; Sultz, H.A.; et al.: Management after myocardial infarction: A controlled trial of the effect of group psychology. J. Psychiat. Med. 5: 253–268 (1974).

40 Rahe, R.; Ward, J.; Hayes, V.: Brief group therapy in myocardial infarction rehabilitation. Three to four year follow-up of controlled trial. Psychosom. Med. 41: 229–242 (1979).

41 Gundle, M.J.; Reeves, B.B., Jr.; Tate, S.; et al.: Psychosocial outcome after coronary artery surgery. Am. J. Psych. 137: 1591–1594 (1980).

42 Jenkins, C.D.; Stanton, B.A.; Savageau, J.A.; et al.: Physical, psychological, social and economic outcomes six months after coronary artery bypass surgery. J. Am. Med. Ass. (in press).

43 Zyzanski, S.J.; Rouse, B.A.; Stanton, B.A.; et al.: Employment changes among patients following coronary bypass surgery: social, medical and psychological correlates. Public Health Report 97: 558–5675 (1982).

44 Boulay, F.M.; David, P.B.; Bourassa, M.G.: Strategies for improving the work status of patients after coronary artery bypass surgery. Circ. 66, Supp. III: 43–49 (1982).

45 Danchin, N.; David, P.; Robert, P.; et al.: Employment following aorto-coronary bypass surgery in young patients. Cariol. 69: 41–49 (1982).

46 Morton, J.R.; Tolan, K.M.: Activity level and employment status after coronary artery bypass surgery. Am. J. Surg. 143: 417–420 (1982).

47 Christopherson, L.K.; Lunde, D.T.: Heart transplant donors and their families, in Castelnuovo-Tedesco, eds., Psychiatric aspects of organ donors and their families; pp. 26 (Grune and Stratton, New York 1971).

48 Christopherson, L.K.; Lunde, D.T.: Selection of cardiac Transplant Recipients and Their Subsequent Psycho-social adjustment. Semin. Psychiat. 3: 36 (1971).

49 Kraft, I.A.: Psychiatric complications of cardiac transplantation, in Castelnuovo-Tedesco, eds., Psychiatric aspects or organ transplantation; pp. 58 (Grune and Stratton, New York 1971).

50 Berenson, C.K.; Grosser, B.I.: Total artificial heart implantation. Arch. Gen. Psychiatr. 41: 910–916 (1984).

Stanley Heller, MD, College of Physicians and Surgeons at Columbia University, St. Luke Roosevelt Hospital, New York, NY 10019 (USA)

Adv. psychosom. Med., vol. 15, pp. 140–166 (Karger, Basel 1986)

Surgical Treatment of Obesity

Albert J. Stunkard, Gary D. Foster, Richard F. Grossman

University of Pennsylvania, School of Medicine, Philadelphia, Pa., USA

The relationship of surgery to obesity is different from that of surgery for many conditions discussed in this volume. Considerable psychological distress often occurs following surgical efforts such as limb amputation, mastectomy, and hysterectomy. In the case of obesity, by contrast, it is the disorder itself that has the untoward psychological and social effects. And the consequences of surgery are, to a surprising degree, benign ones.

This happy circumstance must be qualified at once. Surgical treatment of obesity should be confined solely to persons suffering from severe obesity – those 100% or more above the desireable weights listed in the standard height/weight tables [1]. Thus, this chapter deals with the extremes of obesity. Let us begin, therefore, by attempting to define obesity, and morbid obesity.

Description of Obesity

Obesity is a disorder characterized by excessive accumulation of body fat. A body weight 20% over that given in standard height weight tables [1] is arbitrarily considered obesity. Except for heavily muscled persons, this presumption is usually correct.

Obesity is not a condition for which a precise definition is particularly useful. Unlike many 'real' diseases (and like hypertension) obesity represents one arm of a distribution curve of body fat or body weight, with no sharp cutoff point. Its importance lies in the many, often serious, complications to which obese people are subject. Although the cause of obesity – consuming

Table I. Classification of obesity

Type	Mild	Moderate	Severe
Percentage overweight	40 %	40–100 %	100 %
Prevalence (among obese women)	90.5 %	9.0 %	0.5 %
Pathology	hypertrophic	hypertrophic hyperplastic	hypertrophic hyperplastic
Complications	uncertain	conditional	severe
Treatment	behavior therapy (lay)	diet & behavior therapy (medical)	surgical

more calories than are expended as energy – is a simple one, the factors determining this unbalanced energy equation are varied and complex. Social, psychologic, genetic, developmental, endocrine, exercise, and organic factors have all, to a greater or lesser degree, been implicated. Since a review of all these factors is beyond the scope of this chapter, the interested reader is referred to *Obesity* [2] for a detailed coverage of these topics.

Garrow in England [3] and *Stunkard* in the USA [4] have recently proposed a classification of obesity that is achieving increasing acceptance (table I). It consists of 3 simple categories: mild; moderate; and severe, representing respectively, less than 40% overweight, 41–100% overweight and more than 100% overweight. Surgical treatments is reserved for persons in the severe category; for many of them it is the treatment of choice.

Approximately 0.5% of the female obese population is severely obese, and the percentage of men is probably similar although accurate statistics are lacking [5]. The adipose tissue of severely obese persons is usually both hypertrophic (increased size of fat cells) and hyperplastic (increased number of fat cells). Severe obesity is the one form which presents unequivocal medical complications in almost every person who suffers from it. Treatment for severe obesity has included gastric or intestinal bypass surgery, jaw wiring, vagotomy and a host of more conservative treatments such as fad diets, appetite suppressant medication, and therapeutic starvation. The most successful of these procedures is gastric bypass surgery.

Rationale for a Surgical Approach

The rationale for a surgical approach to the treatment of severe obesity is based upon 3 considerations: 1) severely obese persons have higher rates of mortality and morbidity than their lean counterparts; 2) some obese persons are subject to psychological disturbances specifically related to their obesity and 3) conservative treatment of severe obesity is generally ineffective in causing or maintaining significant weight losses.

Mortality and Morbidity with Severe Obesity

It is clear that above 40% overweight, mortality increases as body weight increases. Three studies [6–8] examining the relationship between body weight and life expectancy in persons less than 60% overweight suggested that, for the morbidly obese, there is an increased risk for premature death (figure 1). A study of severely obese men confirmed this suggestion. *Drenick* et al. [9] calculated the mortality rate for 200 morbidly obese men. For morbidly obese men aged 25–34 years, the death rate was 12 times higher than for men in the general population. This dramatic difference decreased with age, falling to 6 times in the 35–44 year old range and 3 times in the group of 45–54 year olds.

Morbidity, as well as mortality, is strongly related to body weight. For many years it had been believed that this relationship was a linear one and that 'the thinner the better'. More recently *Andres* [10, 11] challenged this belief with evidence that morbidity is highest at both extremes of the body weight distribution and that mild obesity is not associated with increased risk. Even more recently, however, *Garrison* et al. [12] have challenged *Andres'* views by demonstrating that the risk associated with smoking has confounded the relationship between body weight and morbidity. For smoking not only lowers body weight but also confers an increased risk. These investigators have provided new support for the old 'the thinner the better' views, as long as the thinness is not due to smoking. But until other studies are reanalyzed, removing the effect of smoking on morbidity, the association between morbidity and mild obesity remains unclear.

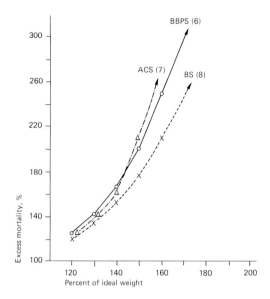

Fig. 1. Acceleration of excess mortality among men and women as their degree of over-weight increases. The segments of lines beyond 140% of average weight in the ACS study [7] and beyond 160% in the Build and Blood Pressure Study (BBPS) [6] and the Build Study (BS) [8] are extrapolations. [From *Van Itallie*. 33.]

Despite the uncertainly about milder forms of obesity, it is clear that more than 40% overweight is associated with increased morbidity. Three serious illnesses, all of which are also potent risk factors for coronary artery disease (hypertension, type II diabetes mellitus, and the hyperlipidemias) are far more prevalent among obese than lean persons [13]. The relationship between obesity and cardiovascular disease is so pronounced that *Kannel and Gordon* assert that 'correction of overweight is probably the most important hygienic measure (aside from avoidance of cigarettes) available for the control of cardiovascular disease' [13]. Furthermore, hypertension, diabetes, and the hyperlipidemias are ameliorated with weight reduction, suggesting that obesity plays a role in their genesis. In addition, some serious disorders are unique to severe obesity, such as the compromised pulmonary function of the *Pickwickian* syndrome [14]. Finally, there is growing evidence that severe obesity, particularly when associated with hypertrophic adipose tissue cells, stimulates proliferation of more adipose tissue cells and increases the severity

Table II. Some conditions associated with morbid obesity

High risk of coronary disease
  Increased mortality associated with myocardial
  infarction
Hypertension (exacerbated by increasing obesity)
Diabetes mellitus (exacerbated by enlarging adipocytes)
Gallbladder disease
Cardiorespiratory dysfunction
  Hypervolemia
  Increased left ventricular filling pressure
  Obesity hypoventilation syndrome*
  Cor pulmonale
  Circulatory congestion
Osteoarthritis of weight-bearing joints
  Particularly knees and back
Psychosocial incapacity
Thromboembolic disease with pulmonary emboli
Operative risks
  Anesthesia and operation more dangerous
  Pulmonary functions compromised
  Increased risk of:
    Wound infection
    Wound dehiscence
    Late hernia formation
    Thrombophlebitis and pulmonary embolism
Thrombosis of the renal veins and vena cava
  Nephrotic syndrome
Cardiomegaly
Abnormalities of liver function and morphology
Uterine fibroid and carcinoma of endometrium
Venous stasis in lower extremities
  Stasis ulcers
  Thrombophlebitis and pulmonary embolism
Interference with diagnosis of:
    Breast cancer
    Ovarian tumor
    Mediastinal masses (sometimes confused with mediastinal lipomatosis)

* Obstructive sleep apnea is a separate syndrome that can occur in mild obesity.

of the obesity [15]. A summary of the conditions associated with severe obesity is provided in table II.

Psychological Disturbances

The second reason for a surgical approach to the treatment of severe obesity is that some obese persons are subject to psychological disorders that are specifically related to their overweight. Contrary to popular belief, the obese population as a whole manifests no more psychopathology than do nonobese populations [16–18]. Two studies have confirmed these findings with morbidly obese persons [19, 20]. However, 2 types of emotional disturbance *are* specifically related to obesity. The first is an untoward emotional response to dieting; the second is a disturbance in body image.

Many obese persons suffer emotional disturbances during efforts at weight reduction [21]. These disturbances are one of the reasons that outpatient treatment of obesity typically has a high attrition rate [4, 22]. The first systematic study of this problem [23] demonstrated that half of all patients had at least one symptom that they attributed to dieting. Other studies have reported similar findings [24]. A review of the literature [21] has established the high incidence of emotional symptoms in both outpatients and inpatients treated for obesity. A study that will be described later, in greater detail [25], showed that morbidly obese persons probably suffer even more severely during dieting than do less obese persons.

The second form of emotional disturbance specific to obese persons is disparagement of the body image [26, 27]. Obese persons with this disturbance characteristically feel that their bodies are grotesque and loathesome and that others view them with hostility and contempt. This feeling is closely associated with self-consciousness and impaired social functioning. It might seem reasonable to suppose that all obese persons have derogatory feelings about their bodies. Such is not the case. Emotionally healthy obese persons have no body image disturbances; in fact, only a minority of neurotic obese persons have such disturbances. Body image disturbances are confined to those who have been obese since childhood; even among these juvenile-onset obese persons, fewer than half suffer from it. But in the group with body image disturbances, neurosis is closely related to obesity, and this group contains a majority of obese persons with specific eating disorders. (Body image issues are discussed further on p. 84 on aesthetic facial surgery and on p. 200 on psychological sequelae of limb amputation.)

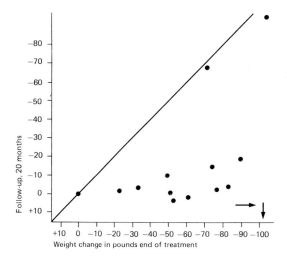

Fig. 2. Figure plotted from data published in *Swanson and Dinello* [32]. See text for explanation of method. Note consistency with which weight is regained.

Failure of Conservative Treatment

The third rationale for a surgical approach to the treatment of severe obesity is the relative failure of more conservative types of treatment. What was stated some years ago is still the case today: most obese persons will not participate in outpatient treatment, those who do will not lose a significant amount of weight and most of those who do lose will regain it [28]. Furthermore, as we have noted, the most common remedy for obesity – dieting – may precipitate emotional disturbance [21]. Although the effectiveness of treatment of all types of obesity is limited, that of morbid obesity is more so. Even the best of conservative approaches [29, 30] results in an average weight loss of no more than 0.7 kg per week. Therefore, in a 6 month program, longer than most, a morbidly obese person would lose only 17 kg. Such a loss is of little evident clinical utility to someone who is more than 45 kg overweight.

Not only do severely obese people have great difficulty losing weight, they have even greater difficulty maintaining weight losses. *Johnson and Drenick* [31] reported that 50% of 121 patients had regained their lost weight within 2–3 years; and by 9 years, 90% were at or above their pretreatment weights. In an even more dramatic demonstration, *Swanson and Dinello* [32] described 25 severely obese patients who were therapeutically starved for an average of 38 days. Within one year, 56% had regained or exceeded their pretreatment weight. Figure 2 shows the poor rate of maintenance among these patients. Points along the diagonal line represent perfect maintenance of weight loss, the points above the diagonal represent additional losses after treatment and the points below the diagonal represent a regain of weight lost during treatment. Note the large number of data points far below the main diagonal. The results of these 2 studies are probably even worse than they appear due to the number of people who did not respond (58% in *Johnson and Drenick*, 28% in *Swanson and Dinello)*, presumably because of a poor treatment outcome. These dismal results have resulted in the strong conclusion of a recent NIH consensus conference: 'The conventional modalities of outpatient treatment for obesity ... have little or nothing to offer the majority of morbidly obese patients, either singly or in combination.' [33]

Intestinal Bypass

When we consider the social and emotional consequences of surgery for obesity, we face a curious paradox. At the present time, because of its far fewer medical complications, gastric bypass surgery has largely supplanted intestinal bypass surgery as the treatment of choice for severe obesity. Yet because of the far larger experience with intestinal bypass, much more is known about the social and emotional consequences of this form of surgery than is known about these consequences of gastric bypass surgery.

One fortunate aspect of the problem created by this paradox is that the social and emotional consequences of the 2 forms of surgery appear to be similar. Accordingly, we will describe these consequences of intestinal bypass surgery in some detail while cautioning the reader that this form of treatment is in rapid decline. It is our expectation and the section on the results of gastric bypass surgery will show that this expectation is a reasonable one, that the kinds of social and emotional consequences observed with intestinal bypass will also be found with gastric bypass.

Intestinal bypass surgery is a basically simple procedure in which 14 inches of proximal jejunum are anastomosed to 4 inches of terminal ileum. The original rationale for this operation was to drastically reduce the absorptive surface of the small intestine and thus to limit the amount of food that could be absorbed. It has since been learned that this mechanism accounts for no more than 25% of the caloric deficit following surgery and that 75%

of the deficit is contributed by a decrease in food intake [34, 35]. There are 2 types of intestinal bypass, the original end-to-side procedure devised by *Payne* [36] and the more recent end-to-end procedure of *Scott* [37]. *Bray* et al. report that the results of the 2 methods are comparable [38–40].

Intestinal bypass surgery produces weight losses that range from 14 kg to more than 100 kg depending upon the length of the intestine left in circuit and the patient's initial weight. Weight is lost in a characteristic pattern, very rapidly at first, and then slowing down to reach a plateau by the end of the second post-operative year. About half of the weight loss occurs during the first 6 months and half of the remaining weight loss during the next 6 months. Less than 25% of the weight loss is lean body mass, which is regained by the third post-operative year [41].

A number of benefits accrue from such marked weight loss and they tend to persist. Glucose intolerance is usually markedly improved and almost all patients are able to discontinue antidiabetic medication. Similarly, hypertension, which is common among severely obese persons, is controlled in the vast majority following surgery and many who required antihypertensive medication can discontinue it. Blood lipid levels decrease, cardiac and pulmonary disease lessen and venous insufficiency and stasis ulcers usually heal [42]. These several benefits provided a strong rationale for the use of intestinal bypass surgery for severe obesity and if more effective forms of treatment had not emerged, it might still be in widespread use. Nevertheless, from the beginning there were obviously serious problems with this form of treatment.

Intestinal bypass is plagued with many severe side reactions. Mortality averages 3%, with a range of from less than 2% to more than 10% [43]. The lowest rates have occured in medical centers which specialize in this form of treatment and where teams of surgeons, internists and psychiatrists were prepared to carry out long-term supportive therapy. Indeed, in the absence of such long-term therapy there have been so many problems that it has been argued that the operation should be permitted only in institutions which have made a commitment to long-term care.

One of the first problems to be noted was liver failure, which was fatal in 1% of patients and which could be reversed only by reoperation to restore intestinal continuity. More recently *Hocking* et al. have reported the development of progressive liver abnormalities, including cirrhosis, up to 5 years post-operatively in as many as 29% of patients [42]. Serious early complications include wound dehiscence, electrolyte imbalance and pulmonary embolus. Patients may later develop urinary calculi, protein deficiency, arthralgia, encephalopathy, renal failure, and a variety of related disorders

[36, 41–44]. Diarrhea and foul-smelling flatus constitute the major complaint of patients, although they decrease after time. *Mills and Stunkard* [35] reported an average rate of 17 stools per day at one month that fell to 4.7 stools per day at 37 months. *Hocking* et al. reported that 72% of their patients had more than 3 bowel movements a day one year after surgery [42]. Clearly this high rate of complications meant that intestinal bypass surgery was warranted only if the alternatives were equally grim and insured that any new form of treatment that produced fewer complications would rapidly supplant it. Such a treatment is gastric bypass and, as expected, it has largely supplanted intestinal bypass surgery.

Psychosocial Outcome of Intestinal Bypass Surgery

Intestinal bypass surgery improves the psychosocial functioning of severely obese patients [45–50]. This finding, reported in the first psychological assessment of bypass patients by *Solow* et al. in 1974 [50] has been the subject of a remarkable degree of consensus in subsequent reports. In that landmark report, *Solow* et al. noted improvement in mood, self-esteem, interpersonal and vocational effectiveness, body image and activity levels and decreased use of denial. This favorable impression is shared by patients, most of whom report satisfaction with the outcome of the surgery [50]. In fact, 80% of the patients in one study indicated that they would not, even in the face of severe somatic complications, have the procedure reversed if it meant a return to severe obesity [51].

Many of the psychosocial benefits of weight loss from surgery are direct results of increased mobility and stamina [47, 52, 53] which, coupled with diminishing self-consciousness [49], encouraged patients to explore social and vocational activities formerly impossible for them. Being able to pass through supermarket and subway turnstiles, ride in public transportation, and fit into theater seats makes a powerful impression on people who had formerly been denied these activities. Their mood improves [49] and their belief in their capacities increases [51]. Patients whose embarrassment and immobility had prevented them from seeking or holding a job have reported successful employment, while people who had been employed reported 'increased productiveness, income and job satisfaction' [52]. Other patients reported starting school 2 and 3 years post-operatively [47, 49]. Occupational gains are long-lived and tend not to be lost by mild or moderate somatic complications [45].

Assertiveness and self-confidence increase after surgery when compared to the patients' typical pre-operative condition of passive-dependency and self-denigration [45–50, 52, 54]. Newly found autonomy is reflected by the frequency with which patients change previously unsatisfactory jobs and homes [47, 52]. *Solow* reported that a majority of patients 3 years after surgery felt 'greater confidence in their own resources, ... reduction in resignation and in a self-reinforcing sense of entrapment, and escape from a chronic sense of helplessness, hopelessness, and unrelieved failure' [48, 49].

One favorable effect of intestinal bypass surgery that occurs relatively early is a diminution in the intensity of body image disparagement, which has been described earlier. This disorder rarely remits spontaneously. Accordingly, it is noteworthy that within a year patients begin to report more positive evaluations of their bodies, even when substantial overweight remains [47, 48]. Some feelings of physical unattractiveness, of course, may remain for 2 years or longer [47, 57], but the overall affective response to body image after the patients' weight has stabilized is strongly positive [48].

Sexual and Marital Relations

Sexual and marital relations are particularly responsive to the effects of weight loss following surgery. A number of reports note that the improvement in self-regard has a particularly favorable effect in increasing both the frequency of sexual relations and the satisfaction with which they are regarded [48, 49, 52]. 61% of one series of patients reported that sex had become more enjoyable [57]. Both fantasies and sexual affairs increase [47, 52]. Consonant with improvements in psychosexual functioning is the awakening among women patients of attentiveness to such aspects of style as lipstick, facial make-up, and fashionable dresses [47].

One quantifiable measure of the psychosocial outcome of intestinal bypass is marital function. Early reports noted tension in marriages arising from the patients' increased self-assertiveness and their assumption of a broad range of new social roles [47, 52]. One such study attracted considerable attention with its report that surgery for morbid obesity exacerbated marital discord and often led to divorce [56]. An elegant study by *Rand* et al. [57] put this finding into perspective. They found that surgery usually had a positive effect on marital relationships even though there was a high rate of divorce. The use of a carefully constructed control group in this study helped to explain the apparent paradox. For it showed that among non-obese persons, as well as among obese ones, conflicted marriages tended to end in divorce and unconflicted marriages tended to endure. Severely obese persons had a higher rate of conflicted marriages than non-obese persons; it was this high rate of conflicted marriages, rather than the surgery, that accounted for their higher rate of divorce. *Rand* et al. interpreted divorce by obese persons as an indication of improved psychological functioning, which made it possible for patients to leave unhappy marriages with spouses who were exploiting them. The experience of one of us (AJS) strongly supports this interpretation of divorce following surgery. Regarding unconflicted marriages, *Rand* et al. note an unequivocal improvement, with both patients and spouses reporting an increase in the frequency of sexual relations and in spouse appraisal of the patient as sexually attractive [57].

Psychobiological Outcome

As striking as are the reports of the psychosocial benefits of intestinal bypass surgery, they have almost certainly underestimated these benefits. For they used an inappropriate control period for comparison with emotional status after surgery; the emotional status just before surgery. The appropriate control period is *not* the period just before surgery, but previous periods when the patient was losing weight without surgery. As noted above, 50% of persons receiving standard medical treatment for obesity experience untoward emotional responses, particularly anxiety and depression [21]. Among morbidly obese persons, furthermore, the incidence of untoward reactions is even higher and they are even more severe [25].

In contrast to these high rates of emotional disturbance during weight loss by medical treatment, *Mills and Stunkard* [35] found that weight loss following intestinal bypass surgery was associated with very little emotional disturbance. Following such surgery there was far less depression, anxiety, irritability and preoccupation with food. Furthermore, half the patients reported an increase in positive emotions such as elation and self-confidence, in sharp contrast to the few who had reported such emotions during dieting.

Changes in eating patterns following surgery were as striking as the changed emotional responses [35]. Before surgery most patients reported highly variable patterns of excessive food intake. After surgery there was a marked decrease in binge-eating, night-eating and snacking, less difficulty in stopping eating, fewer and smaller meals, and rapid weight loss. Patients who did not start eating until later in the day reported a return of appetite for breakfast! As striking as the changes in eating patterns was the fact that they occurred without any voluntary effort on the part of the patients.

These findings have been confirmed by *Bray* et al. who compared the effects of dieting with those of intestinal bypass surgery in a group of severely obese patients on a metabolic ward [34]. During one month on an 800 calorie diet these patients became depressed; intestinal bypass surgery relieved the depression. Following surgery the levels of 3 agents, all linked to satiety, were elevated – enteroglucagon, pancreatic polypeptide and glycerol. Finally, these patients reported a decrease in their preference for highly concentrated sucrose solutions.

These findings suggest that intestinal bypass surgery has produced a major change in the biology of obese persons. What kind of biological change could produce such profound changes in behavior? We have suggested that the surgery lowers a set point around which body weight is regulated [35]. We will return to this issue when we consider gastric bypass surgery for obesity.

The Question of Psychological Ill-Effects

A few early reports of psychiatric assessment of intestinal bypass surgery attributed psychological problems to the surgery [52, 54, 58, 59]. It appears that most of these problems antedated the surgery or stemmed from the physical complications of it. There is now agreement that intestinal bypass is usually followed by improved psychological functioning. This impression is greatly strengthened by the few long-term follow-up studies. Six years after surgery, assessments by both *Solow* et al. [48] and *Castelnuovo-Tedesco* et al. [45] indicated that the psychosocial benefits of intestinal bypass were permanent.

Gastric Bypass

Surgical Procedures and Post-Operative Complications

Gastric bypass has now become the most widely performed surgery for obesity. Its rationale is radical reduction of the amount of food that can be consumed at any one time. In this respect the gastric procedure differs from the intestinal, which permits patients to eat as much as they desire, provided they are willing to tolerate diarrhea [40]. Gastric bypass for treatment of morbid obesity was introduced in 1967 by *Mason*, who was the first to note that obese patients who had undergone the venerable *Billroth II* procedure for peptic ulcer lost large amounts of weight [60]. Gastric bypass, of which there are now several variations, involves establishment of a fundic pouch of approximately 30 ml in size, leaving the remainder of the stomach as a blind pouch attached to the duodenum.

Compared to intestinal bypass, the complications of gastric bypass are fewer and less severe. Were it not for the technical difficulty of performing the gastric operation, it might well have superseded jejunoileal bypass long ago. Complications include anastomotic leak, puncture of the stoma, stomal ulcer, and, before patients become accustomed to their extremely limited stomach capacity, nausea and vomiting following eating.

The Last Word – Vertical Banded Gastroplasty

During the past three years, and with stunning speed, a new gastric reduction procedure has achieved increasing popularity for obesity and is now widely considered the ideal operation [69, 70]. It is vertical banded gastroplasty which consists of a 30 ml vertical pouch oriented along the lesser curvature of the stomach. To provide additional support for the stoma a 1.5 cm wide plastic mesh collar is sewn around the outside of the stomach wall where it is quickly surrounded by connective tissue.

One reason for the rapid success of this operation is that it incorporates the lessons learned from 17 years of experience with gastric procedures. The procedure is far simpler technically than other gastric reduction procedures and it preserves a normal sequence in the passage of food. Location of the pouch along lesser curvature takes advantage of the greater muscle strength of this region and decreases the tendency toward distention that has plagued traditional pouches located in the fundus. Finally, reinforcement of the stoma with a plastic collar greatly decreases the incidence of stomal dilatation that occurred with other gastric reduction procedures.

The results achieved to date support the favorable expectations of vertical banded gastroplasty that had been aroused by the above theoretical issues. The *Iowa group* reports that operative time has been cut by 2/3 with a reduction in the rate of operative mortality to less than 1% and of wound infections to 2.7%, together with virtual elimination of perforation and peritonitis [70]. The weight losses of the *Iowa group's* patients at both 1 and 2 years post-operatively are the equal of those that they had achieved in their extensive experience with gastric bypass. Finally, their revision rate during the first year following surgery has been less than 3%, significantly lower than that of other procedures. *Buckwalter,* a distinguished academic surgeon, has had similar, favorable experience with vertical banded gastroplasty [71].

The recency of vertical banded gastroplasty means that there have been no studies of its psychosocial consequences. The great similarity in the consequences of 2 such dissimilar procedures as intestinal bypass and gastric bypass, however, strongly suggests that the consequences of this relatively minor variant of gastric bypass should be as favorable as those of its predecessor procedures.

Weight Loss

Weight is lost following gastric bypass according to the same pattern as that following intestinal bypass – rapid at first with a slowly decreasing rate over about 2 years. One year after the surgery, the average weight loss ranges from 40–50 kg with a decrease in excess weight of 35–45% [40, 61–63]. Although jejunoileal bypass produces a somewhat larger weight loss, the difference is not clinically significant [61–63].

Psychosocial Outcome

Although the psychosocial effects of gastric bypass have not been studied as widely as those of intestinal bypass, they seem to be just as favorable. The first report to examine the emotional responses to gastric bypass showed the same positive outcome, particularly when the responses were compared, as they should be, to those during previous periods when the patient was losing weight by medical treatment [25]. Figure 3 shows the responses of 80 severely obese patients to weight loss by medical treatment. Severe depressive reactions were experienced by 15% and moderately severe depression by another 26%. Only a minority of the patients had not experienced some degree of depression during earlier attempts at weight loss and even fewer reported no anxiety, irritability or preoccupation with food.

By contrast, the emotional response of these patients to gastric bypass surgery was far more benign, even though they were losing far more weight than in their earlier efforts. Figure 4 shows that about half the patients

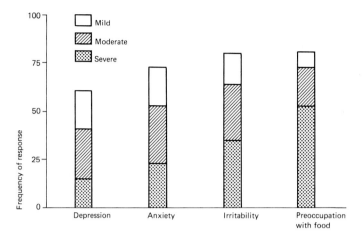

Fig. 3. Untoward responses to previous weight loss by dieting. The percentage of patients who reported severe, moderate, and mild symptoms are indicated on the bars representing depression, anxiety, irritability and preoccupation with food. Only a minority of patients reported no symptoms. (Figure drawn from data in *Halmi, Stunkard, and Mason* [25], by permission.)

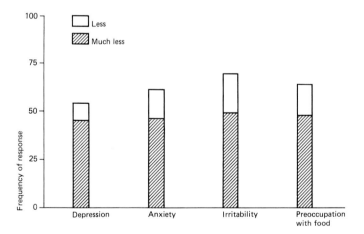

Fig. 4. Comparison of untoward response after gastric bypass with those during dieting. The percentage of patients reporting differences in untoward responses to weight loss after gastric bypass compared to those during dieting. Nearly half reported that their symptoms were much less severe after surgery, and very few reported that they were more severe. (Figure drawn from data in *Halmi, Stunkard, and Mason* [25].)

Table III. Body image disparagement

	Severe	Mild	Absent
Before	70	18	11
After	4	48	45

reported 'much less' dysphoric mood following bypass surgery and another 5–15% reported 'less' dysphoria.

The psychosocial benefits of gastric bypass surgery were not confined to a lessening of negative emotions. Half of the patients reported 'much more' elation and self confidence and 75% reported 'much more' feelings of well-being.

Body image disparagement was also affected by surgery. Before surgery, 70% of patients reported severe body image disparagement and only 11% reported its absence. By contrast, no more than 4% reported severe disparagement after surgery and nearly half were symptom free (table III). One objective measure of body image disparagement is 'mirror avoidance'. Most persons with body image disparagement distinctly dislike looking at themselves in the mirror and may go to great lengths to avoid, even inadvertent, glimpses of themselves, as in store windows [64]. One half of the patients had reported mirror avoidance prior to surgery. 84% of these patients reported that this problem had become less severe, and fully half reported that it was 'much less severe'. Approximately the same proportion (81%) reported they felt 'more desirable' after surgery.

A noteable aspect of these changes in body image was that they were present within 6 months after surgery, at a time when weight loss averaged 31 kg. Pre-operative weight averaged 127 kg. Thus, this profound decrease in body image disparagement occurred when these patients – mostly women – weighted an average of 96 kg.

Two symptoms that deserve special attention are weakness and fatigue. Neither symptom was as frequent as the other untoward emotional reactions during diets in the past. Although they occurred less frequently after surgery than during dieting, the difference was modest. Only a small minority of patients reported that these symptoms had been 'severe' during weight reduction by dietary means, and only 29% reported that were 'much less' during weight reduction by surgical means.

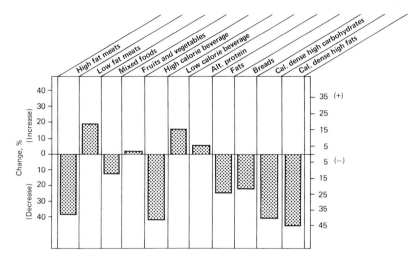

Fig. 5. Changes in the frequency of eating of the different food categories. Increased frequency of consumption is depicted above the 0 line, decreased frequency of consumption below it. Note marked decrease in frequency of consumption of high density fats, high density carbohydrates, high calorie beverages and high fat meats. There are few instances of greater frequency of consumption and all are in the low calorie density categories. (From *Halmi, Mason, Falk, and Stunkard* [65], by permission).

Changes in Eating Behavior

Favorable changes in eating behavior also follow gastric bypass surgery. One such change occurred with satiety. Before surgery 91% of the patients reported that it required 'much' willpower to stop eating; after surgery this number fell to 10%. Similarly, when patients were asked how much more they could eat after having finished a meal, there were marked differences. Before surgery 33% said that they could eat another full meal and only 14% said that they could not eat any more. After surgery only 1% could eat a full meal and 94% could eat no more. These differences are more remarkable in light of what a full meal meant before and after the surgery – a liter or more before surgery and only 50 ml after it!

Another striking change in eating behavior following gastric bypass surgery occurred in the area of food preferences [65]. 50% of the patients reported that high density fat and high density carbohydrates were no longer enjoyable, with smaller percentages reporting a lack of enjoyment of high fat meats and high calorie beverages. The development of dislikes for these foods was highly correlated with decrease in the frequency with which they were consumed ($r = .687$, $p < .05$). The changes in frequency of eating various food types is illustrated in figure 5. In this figure, increased frequency of consumption is depicted above the zero line and decreased frequency of consumption below it. As might be expected from reports of foods no longer found enjoyable, patients also reported a marked decrease in frequency of consumption of high density fats, high density carbohydrates, high calorie beverages and high fat meats. An added measure of the reliability of these responses is the high correlation ($r = .865$, $p < .01$) between changes in the frequency of eating various types of food and reports of reductions in food intake.

This surprising series of changes in behavior following gastric bypass does not exhaust the list. Changes in eating patterns of a similar striking nature have been observed by clinicians although they have not been investigated systematically.

A Theory of Action Concerning Surgery for Morbid Obesity

The changes following gastric bypass precisely parallel those that have been reported after intestinal bypass surgery. Those changes were so profound as to suggest that they derive from major changes in the biology of the organism. Specifically, they suggest that both forms of surgery act by lowering a set point around which body weight is regulated. The idea that body weight is regulated, as opposed to being the passive result of a number of unrelated influences, is relatively new, but the evidence supporting it is strong. Much of this evidence is derived from study of the weight changes after hypothalamic lesions. Traditional explanations of these weight changes had viewed them as simple consequences of overeating or undereating. Animals with ventromedial or lateral hypothalamic lesions become fat or thin, respectively, it was held, because they eat too much or too little. Newer explanations reverse this sequence: such animals overeat or undereat in order to become fat or thin [66]. The target weight they are seeking by their eating behavior (and by metabolic changes) is determined by an alteration in the set point about which their body weight is regulated. Hypothalamic lesions thus affect a physiological regulation and not a single behavior.

Two reports of intestinal bypass surgery of genetically obese [67] and of hypothalamically obese [68] rats provide strong evidence that surgery acts to lower a set point for the regulation of body weight. If this mechanism also accounts for the effect of intestinal bypass surgery in humans it would explain how obese persons can lose weight without special effort. For in this case physiological regulation would support a lowered food intake, rather than opposing it, as during dieting. And persons who eat less in the service of a physiological regulation may have less emotional difficulty than those who eat less in opposition to that regulation. If the effects of gastric bypass surgery so closely parallel those of intestinal bypass surgery, it would seem reasonable that the same mechanism of weight loss may also operate following gastric bypass. It, too, may lower a body weight set point. But the operations are quite dissimilar and their results – emptiness of most of the bowel and small stomach capacity – are very different. How such different results might activate such similar mechanisms must remain for the present a mystery, an intriguing legacy of surgery to our understanding of the regulation of body weight.

Selection of Patients for Surgery

In this chapter, we have focused upon the social and emotional sequelae of surgery for obesity and these sequelae are quite favorable. This optimistic view should not, however, obscure the fact these procedures constitute major surgery with all of the associated dangers. Surgery for obesity should not be entered upon lightly, and never for cosmetic reasons or for obesity of less than great severity. Responsible surgeons agree that a prospective patient should 1) be at least 100% or 45 kg above ideal body weight; 2) have a history of repeated failures with traditional, non-surgical techniques; 3) have no detectable endogenous cause of obesity and 4) have no history of alcoholism, drug abuse, or other psychiatric problems that would compromise his/her cooperation [72, 73].

In general, patients aged between 20–50 tolerate the surgery better and have more favorable outcome [40]. Informed consent is essential, and prospective patients should talk with patients who have undergone both successful and non-successful operations. It is also important that patients understand that for some operations (gastric bypass, vagotomy) long term follow-up is limited or lacking. Responsible surgeons should report the success/failure rate at the hospital in which the operation is performed. Finally, the patient should fully understand the drastic change in eating habits that will be necessary and make a commitment to participate in regular and long term follow-up.

Other Types of Surgery

Although the intestinal and gastric bypass operations are the most common and successful, there are 2 other treatments for morbid obesity that may be useful alone (vagotomy), or as a precursor to surgery (jaw-wiring).

Vagotomy

Truncal vagotomy has recently been performed on a small number of morbidly obese persons [74]. Although new in the treatment of severe obesity, vagotomy has been used to treat duodenal ulcer disease for over 50 years. Furthermore, there have been many years of experience in the use of vagotomy in experimental obesity. This procedure predictably reduces the food intake and body weight of hypothalamic obese animals of a variety of species [75–79] although it has little effect on genetic forms of obesity. The animal data, coupled with the findings that humans treated by vagotomy for duodenal ulcer reported little or no feelings of hunger [80], suggested the use of vagotomy as a treatment for severe human obesity [74, 81, 82].

Kral [82] performed vagotomy on 14 severely obese patients and followed them for more than a year (13–37 months). Their mean weight loss was 20 ± 4 kg with a range of 0–52. The patients reported a marked decrease in their level of hunger and found adherence to supervised weight reduction (diet, exercise and group therapy) easier than before the operation.

If these weight losses can be maintained and replicated with larger number of patients, vagotomy may be an effective treatment for severe obesity. Because of its long term use in the treatment of ulcer disease, the complications and side effects of vagotomy are well known and they are far fewer than those following intestinal bypass. (The lesser amount of long-term data on gastric bypass makes it difficult to compare it with vagotomy.) Unlike the bypass procedures, vagotomy is irreversible. At the present time vagotomy must be considered an experimental procedure.

Jaw-wiring

Maxillo-mandibular fixation or jaw-wiring is a standard treatment for jaw fractures. In the treatment of severe obesity, jaw wiring has been used to restrict the intake of solid food while permitting the ingestion of liquid foods. Weight loss typically averages 35 kg over a 9 month period.

Whether or not the wires should be removed periodically is a matter of some controversy. *Wood* [83] has suggested that they be removed after the first month and then again every 6–8 weeks. On the other hand, *Garrow* [84], who introduced the procedure and who has acquired the greatest experience with it, believes that even temporary removal makes adherence to the diet more difficult. His position is supported by reports of high attrition rates when patients have had 'weekend breaks' [83, 85]. Once the wires are removed, most of the weight lost during treatment is regained [86].

Garrow [84] has reported a small series in which patients were fitted with a nylon waist cord following the removal of the wires. The tightly fitted cord provides patients with a form of continuous feedback that enables them to be acutely aware of any significant weight gain. The initial results suggest that those provided with nylon cords regained less weight than those without cords.

Since most patients who have their jaws wired regain most of the lost weight when the wires are removed, it is not an acceptable treatment by itself. It can, however, serve a useful function as a preparation for surgery, and this is its most common current use [84]. One benefit is that jaw-wiring can help patients get accustomed to the dramatic changes in food intake that occur post-operatively. Secondly, the significant weight loss produced by jaw-wiring makes the severely obese patient a better operative risk.

Due to the experimental nature of vagotomy and relative long-term failure of jaw-wiring, there have no systematic investigations of the psychosocial effects of either procedure.

Conclusions

Surgery for obesity is confined to severe (morbid) obesity, characterized by greater than 100% overweight. Such obesity is associated with high rates of mortality and morbidity and with serious psychosocial impairment. Conservative treatment is ineffective.

Under these circumstances intestinal bypass surgery, designed to bypass most of the absorptive surface of the bowel, achieved great popularity as an effective way of producing large weight losses. Although a variety of serious complications has caused intestinal bypass surgery to be largely supplanted by gastric reduction procedures, the social and emotional consequences of this surgery are remarkably benign. The large weight losses (45 kg and more) that follow intestinal bypass usually are associated with greatly increased mobility and stamina together with greater assertiveness and self-confidence. Sexual and marital relations improve and there is marked diminution in the intensity of body image disparagement. Deviant eating patterns decrease and there is considerable normalization of eating patterns. In contrast to the high rates of emotional disturbance during weight loss by dietary treatment, intestinal bypass surgery is usually followed by improved psychosocial functioning.

The many complications of intestinal bypass surgery have led to a variety of gastric reduction procedures, designed to radically reduce the amount of food that can be ingested at any one time. The best studied of these is the gastric bypass introduced in 1967. Intensive experience with this procedure over the subsequent years has revealed fewer complications than with intestinal bypass and it is becoming the most widely used treatment for morbid obesity. Although the psychosocial consequences of gastric bypass surgery have not been studied as extensively a those of intestinal bypass surgery, they appear just as favorable. Patients who had experienced high rates of untoward emotional reactions to weight loss by dieting found their psychological states improving during weight loss following gastric bypass. Disparagement of the body image decreased and patients were far more readily satiated. Food preferences shifted toward items of low caloric density and favorable changes in eating patterns ensued.

These results of 2 different surgical procedures are so profound as to suggest that they derive from a major change in the biology of the organism. Specifically, they suggest that these surgical treatments act by lowering a set point around which body weight is regulated. What began as mechanical efforts to impair the absorption or the ingestion of nutrients has resulted in a promising treatment for a serious disorder and an intriguing means of exploring the most basic psychobiological functions.

References

1   Society of Actuaries, Metropolitan Life Insurance Company. Frequency of overweight and underweight. Stat. Bull. *41:* 4–7 (1960).
2   Stunkard, A.J. (ed.): Obesity (Saunders, Philadelphia 1980).
3   Garrow, J.S.: Treat Obesity Seriously (Churchill Livingston, London 1981).

4   Stunkard, A.J.: The current status of treatment for obesity; in Stunkard, A.J.; Stellar, E.,
     Eating and its disorders, pp. 159–173 (Raven, New York 1984).
5   Obese and overweight adults in the United States. Vital and health statistics. Series 11, No.
     230: DHHS Publication No. 83–1680 (1983).
6   Society of Actuaries: Build and blood pressure studies. 1957. Vol. 1. Chicago (1959).
7   Lew, E.A.; Garfinkel, L.: Variations in mortality by weight among 750,000 men and
     women. J. Chron. Dis. *32:* 563–576 (1979).
8   Society of Actuaries and Association of Life Insurance Medical Directors: Build Study,
     1979. Chicago (in press).
9   Drenick, E.J.; Bale, G.S.; Seltzer, F.; Johnson, D.G.: Excessive mortality and causes of
     death in morbidly obese men. J. Am. Med. Ass. *243:* 443–445 (1980).
10   Andres, R.: Effect of obesity on total mortality. Inter. J. Obes. *4:* 38–386 (1980).
11   Andres, R.: Aging, diabetes and obesity: Standards of normality. Mt. Sinai J. Med. *48:*
     489–495 (1981).
12   Garrison, R.J.; Feinleib, M.; Castelli, W.P.; McNamara, P.M.: Cigarette smoking as a con-
     founder of the relationship between relative weight and long-term mortality. J. Am. Med.
     Ass. *249:* 2199–2203 (1983).
13   Kannel, W.B.; Gordon, T.: Physiological and medical concomitants of obesity: The
     Framingham Study; in Bray, Obesity in America. U.S. Department of Health, Education
     and Welfare. NIH Publication No. 79–359, Washington, D.C., U.S. Government Printing
     Office (1979).
14   Bierman, E.L.: Obesity; in Wyngaarden. J.; Smith, L.H., Cecil Textbook of Medicine; 16th
     ed. (Saunders, Philadelphia 1982).
15   Sjöström, L.: Fat cells and body weight; in Stunkard, A.J., Obesity, pp. 72–100 (Saunders,
     Philadelphia 1980).
16   Crisp, A.J.; McGuiness, B.: Jolly fat: Relation between obesity and psychoneurosis in a
     general population. Brit. Med. J. *1:* 7–9 (1979).
17   Moore, M.E.; Stunkard, A.J.; Srole, L.: Obesity, social class and mental illness. J. Am.
     Med. Assoc. *181:* 962–966 (1962).
18   Silverstone, T.: Psychosocial aspects of obesity. Proc. Roy. Med. Soc. *61:* 371 (1968).
19   Halmi, K.A.; Stunkard, A.J.; Mason, E.E.: Psychiatric diagnosis of morbidly obese gastric
     bypass patients. Am. J. Psychiat. *137:* 470–472 (1980).
20   Holland, J.; Masling, J.; Copely, D.: Mental illness in lower class normal, obese and hyper-
     obese women. Psychosom. Med. *32:* 351–357 (1970).
21   Stunkard, A.J.; Rush, A.J.: Dieting and depression reexamined: A critical review of
     reports of untoward responses during weight reduction for obesity. Ann. Int. Med. *81:*
     526–533 (1974).
22   Volkmar, F.R.; Stunkard, A.J.; Woolston, J.; Bailey, R.A.: High attrition rates in commer-
     cial weight reduction programs. Arch. Int. Med. *141:* 426–428 (1981).
23   Stunkard, A.J.; McLaren-Hume, M.: The results of treatment for obesity. Arch. Int. Med.
     103: 79–85 (1959).
24   Silverstone, J.T.; Lascelles, B.D.: Dieting and depression. Brit. J. Psychiat. *112:* 513–519
     (1966).
25   Halmi, K.A.; Stunkard, A.J.; Mason, E.E.: Emotional responses to weight reduction by
     three methods: gastric bypass, jejunoileal bypass and diet. Am. J. Clin. Nutr. *33:* 446–451
     (1980).
26   Stunkard, A.J.; Mendelson, M.: Obesity and body image: I. Characteristics of disturbances

in the body image of some obese persons. Am. J. Psychiat. *123:* 1296–1300 (1967).

27 Stunkard, A.J.: The pain of obesity, pp. 236 (Bull, Palo Alto 1976).

28 Stunkard, A.J.: From explanation to action in psychosomatic medicine: The case of obesity. Psychosom. Med. *37:* 195–236 (1975).

29 Wing, R.R.; Jeffery, R.W.: Outpatient treatments of obesity: A comparison of methodology and clinical results. Int. J. Obes. *3:* 261–279 (1979).

30 Craighead, L.W.; Stunkard, A.J.; O'Brien, R.: Behavior therapy and pharmacotherapy for obesity. Arch. Gen. Psychiat. *38:* 763–768 (1981).

31 Drenick, E.J.; Johnson, D.: Weight reduction by fasting and semistarvation in morbid obesity: Long-term follow-up. Int. J. Obes. *2:* 123–132 (1978).

32 Swanson, D.W.; Dinello, F.A.: Follow-up of patients starved for obesity. Psychosom. Med. *32:* 209–214 (1970).

33 Van Itallie, T.B.: 'Morbid' obesity: A hazardous disorder the resists conservative treatment. Am. J. Clin. Nutr. *33:* 358–363 (1980).

34 Bray, G.A.; Barry, R.E.; Benfield, J.; Castelnuovo-Tedesco, P.; Rodin, J.: Intestinal bypass surgery for obesity decreases food intake and taste preferences. Am. J. Clin. Nutr. *29:* 779–783 (1976).

35 Mills, M.J.; Stunkard, A.J.: Behavior changes following surgery for obesity. Am. J. Psychiat. *133:* 527–531 (1976).

36 Payne, J.H.; DeWind, L.T.: Surgical treatment of obesity. Am. J. Surg. *118:* 141–147 (1969).

37 Scott, H.W.; Law, D.H.: Clinical appraisal of jejunoileal shunt in patients with morbid obesity. Am. J. Surg. *117:* 246–253 (1969).

38 Bray, G.A.; Faloon, W.W.; Mendeloff, A.I.: Surgical treatment of obesity. Am. Fam. Phys. *15:* 111–113 (1977).

39 MacLean, L.D.: Intestinal bypass operations for obesity: A review. Canad. J. Surg. *19:* 387–399 (1976).

40 Mason, E.E.: Surgical treatment of obesity, pp. 78–136 (Saunders, Philadelphia 1981).

41 Blackburn, G.L.; Miller, M.M.: Surgical Treatment of Obesity; in Conn, H.L.; DeFelice, E.A.; Kuo, P., Health and Obesity, pp. 149–166 (Raven, New York 1983).

42 Hocking, M.P.; Duerson, M.C.; O'Leary, P.; Woodward, E.R.: Jejunoileal bypass for obesity: Late follow-up in 100 cases. N. Engl. J. Med. *17:* 995–999 (1983).

43 Bray, G.A.: Jejunoileal bypass, jaw wiring and vagotomy; in Stunkard, Obesity, pp. 369–387 (Saunders, Philadelphia 1980).

44 Iber, F.L.; Cooper, M.: Jejunoileal bypass for the treatment of massive obesity. Prevalence, morbidity, and short- and long-term consequences. Am. J. Clin. Nutr. *30:* 4–15 (1977).

45 Castelnuovo-Tedesco, P.; Weinberg, J.; Buchanan, D.C.; Scott, H.W.: Long-term outcome of jejunoileal bypass surgery for superobesity: A psychiatric assessment. Am. J. Psychiat. *139:* 1248–1252 (1982).

46 Castelnuovo-Tedesco, P.: Jejunoileal bypass for superobesity. A psychiatric assessment; in Freyberger, Advances in psychosomatic Medicine; vol. 10, pp. 196–206 (S. Karger, Basel 1980).

47 Castelnuovo-Tedesco, P.; Schiebel, D.: Studies of superobesity: II. Psychiatric appraisal of jejunoileal bypass surgery. Am. J. Psychiat. *133:* 26–31 (1976).

48 Solow, C.; Silberfarb, P.M.; Swift, K.: Psychological and behavioral consequences of intestinal bypass; in Bray, G.A., Recent advances in obesity research II. (Newman, London 1978).

49 Solow, C.: Psychosocial aspects of intestinal bypass surgery for massive obesity: Current status. Am. J. Clin. Nutr. *30:* 103–108 (1977).

50 Solow, C.; Silberfarb, P.M.; Swift, K.: Psychosocial effects of intestinal bypass surgery for severe obesity. N. Engl. J. Med. *290:* 300–304 (1974).

51 Faloon, W.W.; Flood, M.S.; Aroesty, S.; Sherman, C.D.: Assessment of jejunoileostomy for obesity – some observations since 1976. Am. J. Clin. Nutr. *33:* 431–439 (1980).

52 Crisp, A.H.; Kalucy, R.S.; Pilkington, T.R.E.; Gazet, J.C.: Some psychological consequences of ileojejunal bypass surgery. Am. J. Clin. Nutr. *30:* 108–120 (1977).

53 Kuldau, J.M.; Rand, C.S.W.: Negative psychiatric sequelae to jejunoileal bypass are often not correlated with operative results. Am. J. Clin. Nutr. *33:* 502–503 (1980).

54 Abram, H.S.; Meixel, S.A.; Webb, W.W.; Scott, H.W.: Psychological adaptation to jejunoileal bypass for morbid obesity. J. Nerv. Ment. Dis. *162:* 151–157 (1976).

55 Silberfarb, P.M.; Phelps, P.J.; Hauri, P.; Solow, C.: Effects of intestinal bypass surgery on body concept. J. Consul. Clin. Psychol. *46:* 1415–1418 (1978).

56 Neill, J.R.; Marshall, J.R.; Yale, C.E.: Marital changes after intestinal bypass surgery. J. Am. Med. Ass. *240:* 447–450 (1978).

57 Rand, C.S.W.; Kuldau, J.M.; Robbins, L.: Surgery for obesity and marriage quality. J. Am. Med. Ass. *247:* 1419–1422 (1982).

58 Espmark, S.: Psychological adjustment before and after bypass surgery for extreme obesity – a preliminary report. Presented at the First International Congress on Obesity (London, October 9–11, 1974).

59 Kalucy, R.S.; Crisp, A.H.: Some psychological and social implications of massive obesity. A study of some psychosocial accompainments of major fat loss occuring without dietary restriction in massively obese patients. J. Psychosom. Res. *18:* 465 (1974).

60 Mason, E.E.; Ito, C.: Gastric bypass in obesity. Surg. Clin. N. Amer. *47:* 1345 (1967).

61 Griffen, W.O.; Young, V.L.; Stevenson, C.C.: A prospective comparison of gastric and jejunoileal bypass procedures for morbid obesity. Ann. Surg. *186:* 500–509 (1977).

62 Buckwalter, J.A.: A prospective comparison of the jejunoileal and gastric bypass operations for morbid obesity. World J. Surg. *1:* 757–768 (1977).

63 Alden, J.F.: Gastric and jejunoileal bypass. Arch. Surg. *112:* 799–806 (1977).

64 Horan, J.J.: Negative covarant probability: an analogue study. Behav. Res. Ther. *12:* 265–267 (1974).

65 Halmi, K.A.; Mason, E.E.; Falk, J.; Stunkard, A.J.: Appetitive behavior after gastric bypass for obesity. Int. J. Obes. *5:* 457–464 (1981).

66 Keesey, R.E.: A set-point analysis of the regulation of body weight; in Stunkard, A.J., Obesity, pp. 144–165 (Saunders, Philadelphia 1980).

67 Kissileff, H.R.; Nakashima, R.K.; Stunkard, A.J.: Effects of jejunoileal bypass on meal patterns in genetically obese and lean rats. Am. J. Physiol. *237:* 217–224 (1979).

68 Sclafani, A.; Koopmans, H.S.; Vaselli, J.R.; Reichman, M.: Effects of intestinal bypass surgery on appetite, food intake, and body weight in obese and lean rats. Am. J. Physiol. *234:* 3389 (1978).

69 Mason, E.E.: Vertical banded gastroplasty for obesity. Ann. Surg. *117:* 701–706 (1982).

70 Mason, E.E.: Vertical banded gastroplasty. Unpublished manuscript. Department of Surgery, University of Iowa (1984).

71 Buckwalter, J.A.: Personal communication. June 3, 1983.

72 Kral, J.G.: Surgical Therapy; In Greenwood, M.R.C. (ed.), Obesity, pp. 25–38 (Churchill Livingstone, New York 1983).

73 Van Itallie, T.B.; Kral, J.G.: Guidelines for surgery for morbid obesity. Council of the American Society for Clinical Nutrition. Am. J. Clin. Nutr. (in press).

74 Kral, J.G.: Effects of truncal vagotomy on body weight and hyperinsulinemia in morbid obesity. Am. J. Clin. Nutr. *33:* 416–419 (1980).

75 Powley, T.L.; Opsahl, C.A.: Ventromedial hypothalamic obesity abolished by subdiaphragmatic vagotomy. Am. J. Physiol. *266:* 25 (1974).

76 Rezek, M.; Vanderweele, D.A.; Novin, D.: Stages in the recovery of feeding following vagotomy in rabbits. Behav. Biol. *14:* 75 (1975).

77 Fox, K.A.; Kipp, S.C.; Vanderweele, D.A.: Dietary self-selection following subdiaphragmatic vagotomy in the white rat. Am. J. Physiol. *231:* 1790 (1976).

78 Mordes, J.P.; Herrera, M.G.; Silen, W.: Decreased weight gain and food intake in vagotomized rats. Proc. Soc. Exptl. Biol. Med. *156:* 257 (1977).

79 Louis-Sylvestre, J.: Feeding and metabolic patterns in rats with truncular vagotomy or with transplanted beta cells. Am. J. Physiol. *235:* 119 (1978).

80 Dragstedt, L.R.; Palmer, W.L.; Schafer, P.W.; Hodges, P.C.: Supra-diaphragmatic section of the vagus nerves in the treatment of duodenal and gastric ulcers. Gastroenter. *3:* 450 (1944).

81 Kral, J.G.: Vagotomy for treatment of severe obesity. Lancet *2:* 307–308 (1978).

82 Kral, J.G.; Gortz, L.: Truncal vagotomy in morbid obesity. Int. J. Obesity *5:* 431–435 (1981).

83 Wood, G.D.: Early results of treatment of the obese by a diet enforced by maxillo-mandibular fixation. J. Oral Surg. *35:* 461 (1977).

84 Garrow, J.S.; Gardiner, G.T.: Maintenance of weight loss in obese patients following jaw wiring. Brit. Med. J. *282:* 858–860 (1981).

85 Castelnuovo-Tedesco, P.; Buchanan, D.C.; Hall, H.D.: Jaw wiring for obesity. Gen. Hosp. Psychiat. *2:* 156–159 (1980).

86 Kark, A.E.: Jaw wiring. Am. J. Clin. Nutr. *33:* 420–424 (1980).

Albert J. Stunkard, MD, University of Pennsylvania, School of Medicine, Philadelphia, PA 19104 (USA)

Adv. psychosom. Med., vol. 15, pp. 167–179 (Karger, Basel 1986)

Renal Transplantation and the New Medical Era

Norman B. Levy

Professor of Psychiatry, Medicine and Surgery, New York Medical College and Director, Liaison Psychiatry Division, Westchester County Medical Center, Valhalla, N.Y., USA

Of all the vital organs, only the kidney can be transplanted by a procedure which is well beyond the experimental stage and has been so for about 2 decades. The use of renal transplantation and artificial kidney dialysis has heralded in a new medical era, one in which diseased organs are replaced rather than treated.

The major problem in transplantation is that of rejection, making transplant surgery heavily dependent upon immunological support and research. Among the most significant recent advancements is the more frequent use of pretransplant blood transfusions [1]. Further improvement is anticipated in the use of HLA-DR-histocompatibility typing [2]. Recently a worldwide study has been completed showing the efficacy of a new immunosuppressant drug called cyclosporin. The U.S. Food and Drug Administration has removed this medicine from the experimental list making it potentially available to all. Although a significant factor inhibiting the use of cyclosporin in its cost, approximately $5,000 per year per person, it may share with other revolutionary drugs such as cortisone and the broad spectrum antibiotics a rapid reduction in its price. On the horizon is the possible use of human monoclonal antibodies to selected T-cell subsets [2].

Renal transplantation exists competitively with other forms of treatment of kidney failure. Its uniqueness centers around the life that a successful transplantation offers: being as close to normality as is possible in kidney failure, even with the side effects of steroids. On the negative side is the perpetual Sword of Damocles that transplant patients experience with the potential of organ rejection. As to different forms of transplantation, for those

younger than 50 years but not very small children, a graft from a histocompatible living related donor gives the best results. In the United States about
30% of all renal transplants are from related donors. However, 60% of patients with newly diagnosed renal failure are over 50 years old and most patients do not have an HLA-compatible donor. The one year rejection rate of
the living related kidneys is 25% and of cadaveric kidneys 39%.

In the United States alone about 10,000 new patients per year are potentially treatable either by renal transplantation or dialysis. In 1983, 65,000
patients were on dialysis. Data from 1984 indicate that 5,000 U.S. patients
had a renal transplantation. Clearly, many more patients were treated by
various forms of dialysis than received transplantation. However with
advances in the immunology of rejection and the greater availability of
cadaveric kidneys, it is anticipated that in the future renal transplantation
will be the usual rather than the less likely form of treatment for kidney
failure [3].

Since the inception of its use as a method of treatment for renal failure
behavioral scientists have been making systematic observations of patients,
undergoing renal transplantation [4–18]. Observations made concerning psychological stresses and methods of handling the stresses of renal transplanta-
tions may be applicable to other methods of artificial organ substitution. In
the oncoming years it is anticipated that the transplantation of the heart, pan-
creas, lungs and liver may no longer be highly selective and experimental but
rather a standard method of treating the failure of these organs. (For further
discussion on cardiac transplantation, refer to p. 124.)

Pre-Operative Issues

Determinants of Method of Treatment

In actual practice, the single and most significant factor dictating
whether or not a patient is seriously considered for a renal transplantation
is the nature of the nephrological center caring for that patient. There is much
regional variation, an example of which is that home dialysis is greatly fa-
vored in the northwest; much less popular in the eastern part of the United
States; and in great disfavor in Europe. The nature of the relationship
between nephrologists and their renal transplantation centers can be a most
significant factor determining whether or not a patient receives a transplantation. Many nephrologists favor that which they know most about. There are

Continious Ambulatory Peritoneal Dialysis (CAPD) nephrologists, home dialysis nephrologists, center peritoneal nephrologists and transplant nephrologists. Although many maintain an eclectic attitude, the great variation of treatments recommended at different centers underscores the fact that the treatment of kidney failure is still in its early phases. The patient with an HLA-compatible related donor stands a better chance to be transplanted than a person who would need a cadaveric kidney. However the search for a histocompatible donor usually only can take place as the result of the direction of a nephrologist with a laboratory capable of doing tissue typing. In addition, there are selfish economic factors which may cause nephrologists to favor continued treatment in their own units rather than to lose their patients to transplant surgeons. Although such individuals are uncommon, unfortunately they are not entirely rare. Even when a transplant is feasible, waiting lists are common; since the availability of related donors, renal transplant surgeons and facilities are all in relatively short supply.

The Transplant Donor

The process by which one is chosen to be a donor can be a curious one. Some patients ask their family members for a kidney. Most others either leave it to an intermediary person such as a renal physician or a family member to ask for them or insist that nobody be asked. Sometimes a 'black sheep' of the family is selected. Here the 'bad' family member is 'punished' by kidney donation surgery by which he or she may receive 'absolution' for sins of the past, enabling reentry into the family, less blemished.

The unconscious motivation of some donors make their gift a method of receiving protection against illness, as a donation to a blind beggar is enhanced by the beggar announcing: 'Thank God you are not blind'. The common denominator in most donations is one of enhancing one's image and self-esteem. Maternal donors often are motivated by the desire that their child experience a 'rebirth' from a life of renal failure to one of normality. In addition to its wish fulfillment, such a donation may have behind it a method of expiation of guilt of having given birth to a defective child.

Another common denominator among kidney donors is one of rescuing the recipient. A mother donated a kidney in the hope that her son would be made strong enough to separate from his ungratifying wife. Another fantasy of both donor and recipient is one of impregnation, in which the donor is seen as having inseminated the recipient.

The decision to donate a kidney is often made without much reflection, according to many clinicians' experience. There is usually little or no conscious deliberation about the meaning of the gift, its inconvenience, pain and the possible disappointment that may be experienced if the graft is rejected. Most kidney donation is spontaneous [18, 26]. In one study, only 3 of 26 donors were directly asked to donate a kidney, the others volunteered themselves [24].

The reality is that the incidence of death from such a donation is exceedingly low. Also, the chances of the donor 'needing' the donated kidney at a later time are restricted to the not-very-likely-possibility that he or she may sustain trauma to the remaining kidney which would render it severely reduced in function or not at all functional.

Donors do experience a good deal of post-operative pain and often post-operative 'blues'. The latter is connected with the change of focus from being a central or near central person pre-operatively to being out of the limelight post-operatively. Disappointment may also result from what donors may perceive as recipient ingratitude, not only because gratitude is not too common a characteristic of people in general but also because the new post-operative priorities make the recipient less aware of the donor. After receiving a kidney, the recipient is pre-occupied with issues of personal survival and kidney survival.

The donation of an organ is an act of intimacy in which there is also a frequent desire to reinstate a pre-existing bond to the recipient. A middle aged woman gave a kidney to her niece in the hope that this would reunite them to the close mother/daughter relationship they had several years before. As preparation for the operation proceeded, the donor saw that the niece was not becoming closer to her than she had been in recent years. By the time of the operation, the frustrated donor said: 'She can take my God damm kidney and I will never talk to her again!'

Probably the most extensive study done of donors was performed by Simmons and her associates of a group of 130 related donors at the University of Minnesota [18]. By the use of a questionnaire study, she found a greater willingness to donate than was assumed either by the lay or medical public. Confirming the impression of others, she found that in the vast majority of cases, the decision to donate was made without much deliberation or without any at all.

Post-transplant, *Simmons* [18] reports the vast majority of donors indicated that they were happy that they made a donation, felt closer to the recipient and experienced greater levels of self-esteem and happiness. However 7%

of recipients and 6% of donors related that they experienced more difficulty after surgery because of the donation. Moreover, 20% of recipients had displeasure at what they perceived as the difficulty in their never being able to pay back the donor for the gift.

One prominent source of donor dissatisfaction in *Simmons'* study [18] occured if the donor was a male, a brother or son of the recipient, especially if married and with one's own family obligations. Those donors who believed that the recipient was not doing well one year post transplant were also less likely to see their donation in a positive way as were those in whom the transplant was rejected. Here however, only 18% of donors of kidneys which were rejected expressed regret. This study points quite positively to the experience of donation with a significant small percentage feeling to the contrary. These findings go counter to *Kemph* who was impressed by the unconscious resentment of donors reporting episodes of depression in donors in the period after transplantation [7].

In general men tend to be more threatened than women in receiving a donation from a member of the opposite sex. Some male recipients experience gender confusion from a donation from recipients of the opposite sex. One male recipient needed to be reassured by his transplant surgeon that the kidney to be donated by a female would not result in his having to sit while urinating. The latter response underscores the fact that the urogenital system is involved in kidney disease and that patients whose gender identify is tenuous may experience gender confusion with a transplant procedure.

Cadaveric Transplants

The major source of kidneys are donated from victims of traumatic deaths. The adage, 'Don't bury your kidneys, recycle them!' has appeal for many people. Most states have instituted a system by which prospective donors, namely all licensed motor vehicle operators, may express their intent to donate body organs on their driver's license. Many factors play a role in determining whether or not an individual who has expressed the desire to donate a kidney and then dies will have the kidneys removed for transplant donation. Among these determinant are: the approval of the donation by the deceased's relatives, the circumstances and nature of the trauma, the availability of a system at the site of death in which potential donors can be identified, and the availability of a mechanism by which kidneys may be harvested and transported to a center with an identified compatible prospective recipient.

The recipient of a cadaveric transplant may have great curiosity about the individual who donated the kidney. Many recipients experience some survival guilt at having reaped advantage from the death of another person. Some recipients shy away from learning anything about the donor lest their guilt be enhanced, but others have great interest in learning more about the donor. Such interest is often quite similar to that of an adopted child toward his biological parents. Accordingly most transplant surgeons respond by giving only minimal identifying data such as sex and approximate age. At times circumstances make the organ's availability public information, such as a disasterous local automobile accident. At times the kidney recipient will incorporate what he or she believes to be the characteristics of the donor. A patient known to the author of this chapter had delusions of being possessed by the transplanted kidney. Such a response underscores the importance of pre-transplant screening out actively psychotic individuals, especially since post-operative use of steroids tends to enhance pre-existing psychotic disorders.

Post-Operative Issues

Psychological Factors and Organ Rejection/Acceptance

The notion that psychological factors may be one of a myriad determinants of organ rejection or acceptance has been an issue of great interest to behavioral scientists, transplant surgeons and nephrologists [6, 15, 16, 19–24]. There are several case reports which deal with this question, but none which answer it. *Eisendrath* reported that 8 of 11 patients who died following renal transplant surgery had experienced panic and a sense of pessimism about their transplantation to a degree not observed in the survivors [6]. *Viederman* reported on a patient in which giving-up was seen as the cause of organ rejection [16]. (P. 23, 'Psychological Intervention with Surgical Patients: Evaluation and Outcome' and p. 124, 'Psychiatric Aspects of Cardiac Surgery' also discuss outcomes related to pre-operative anxiety and depression.) Other reports, not directly answering the question but shedding some light on associated issues, include that of Basch who studied 9 related and 19 cadaveric kidney transplant patients [15]. He found that in live related donors, family conflicts were heightened between donor and recipient because of the transplantation procedure and that recipients of cadaveric kidneys were affected post-operatively by fantasies about the deceased donor and about their own attitudes toward death and dying.

Steinberg et al. studied 26 recipients of kidney transplants at the Downstate Medical Center during the year 1976 [24] and their donor, pre- and post-operatively. Only one recipient was not on hemodialysis while awaiting transplant surgery. All 25 hemodialysis patients were not satisfied with the quality of their life while on hemodialysis and saw transplant surgery as offering them a better opportunity for enjoying life. The interviews of recipients and donors were audio tape recorded, transcribed and studied by the three investigators. All 3, independent from each other, rated the prospective recipients on a scale of 1 to 5, representing a spectrum of predicted rejection or acceptance. The basis of positive evaluation, i.e. for success of the procedure, was the absence of ambivalence toward the surgery and about the donor; realistic expectations concerning the future; reasonable optimism concerning the oncoming operative procedure and the relative lack of serious depressive symptoms. These investigators were unable to show a statistically significant association between their predictions and the actual outcome of surgery. They believed that their difficulties in predicting outcome on psychological data alone include the fact that a great deal of selection occurred presurgically so that those who were less desirable psychosocially were already eliminated by the transplant surgeon. They also thought that the relatively small number, 26, did not permit sufficient statistical separation of the psychological from the many other factors involved in determining failure or success in the procedure.

Despite the inability to predict transplant survival in these medically complicated cases, they made some interesting observations on the lack of realistic expectations on the part of most of the patients. Although some of this lack of realism was due to the use of pre-operative optimism as a coping technique, half of the patients in this study showed a major disparity between reality and their expectations. For example, 6 had no accurate concept of immunosuppressant medications and 7 had no accurate concept of the phenomenon of rejection, although all had been informed of its existence. A common wish fulfilling fantasy held by both recipients and donors was that transplantation would essentially cure the recipients and return them back to the kind of life they had prior to kidney disease. Such a thought was consciously expressed by two patients, both of whom had lupus. The extent of commitment to the procedure seemed quite great on part of donors and recipients alike. At times the extent of commitment required their repressing or failing to learn about its shortcomings. These investigators were impressed that once a commitment was made to transplantation, the educational process is interfered with because of the wish fulfillment involved in the operation. They recommended that kidney recipients be informed early in their treatment about the facts surrounding the surgical procedure such as the chances of success or failure, including both the details of side effects of being on immunosuppressants, and the impact of facing an uncertain future. They believe that otherwise such patients, faced with side effects of medication or with rejection, may become seriously depressed, feeling they have not been treated honestly by their physicians.

Post-Operative Psychiatric Complications

Post-operatively the patient battles for life and against early rejection, putting all other issues in a background position. Having survived the early post-operative course, the patient is presented with some of the side effects of large doses of steroids necessary to protect against organ rejection. The patient experiences changes in appearance with moon facies, acne, possibly a buffalo hump and changes in the distribution of body fat and body contour. Such changes, especially in facial appearance, can be devastating, in particular for the more narcissistic patient. Some may be especially mortified about these changes not only in themselves but also because they produce a common appearance among fellow patients on high doses of steroids: they all tend to look, in a certain way, like each other's siblings.

Concerning the psychological effects of steroids, euphoria can be an early complication, but it is more characteristically replaced by depression or an increase in a pre-existing depression. Psychoses, in particular paranoid psychoses, are not uncommon among patients on high doses of steroids [27]. This may represent a worsening of a pre-existing psychiatric illness or the precipitation of a mini-psychosis in a patient with a borderline personality disorder. The presence of severe depression or psychosis in a patient on high doses of steroids calls for the differential between an illness caused by steroids or other factors. A careful mental status should be performed. Steroids produce no change in intellectual (cognitive) functions, whereas a psychosis connected with organ rejection and uremia or diabetic acidosis will show impairment in recent memory, abstraction and orientation. (For futher discussion of delirium, refer to p. 51.) Whatever the cause of either depression or psychosis, appropriate medication should be used: an antipsychotic in the presence of psychosis and an antidepressant for a major depressive. In addition, the underlying psychosocial issues need to be addressed.

Sexual Functioning in Transplant Patients

Until 12 years ago the sexual problems of renal transplant recipients had not been systematically investigated. Our knowledge base was restricted to case vignettes, chiefly of patients undergoing hemodialysis. The first systematic study of patients undergoing hemodialysis and of recipients of renal transplants was performed by the author of this chapter and reported in 1973 [28]. Questionnaires were sent to the membership of the National Association of Patients on Hemodialysis and Transplantation (NAPHT) asking them about their sexual functions during 3 periods of time: before they were uremic, after being uremic and untreated and since being treated either by dialysis or renal transplantation. Men were questioned concerning the frequency of sexual intercourse and the incidence of impotence. Impotence was defined here as difficulty getting or maintaining an erection for the purpose of sexual intercourse. Women were questioned concerning frequency of sexual intercourse and frequency of orgasm during intercourse. The cooperation of NAPHT was crucial to the success of this study, and indeed, 67% of the 1,167 questionnaires mailed were returned.

The study showed that patients who received successful transplants showed an improvement in their sexual functioning but, for the group as a whole, sexual functioning of transplant patients did not return to the level experienced before the onset of uremia. Of the 56 male transplant patients studied, 24 (43%) were impotent. This contrasts of 59% of the hemodialysis patients who reported being impotent. Of the group of 81 male and 43 female patients who had functional renal grafts or had been transplanted and whose grafts were rejected, 24 men and 8 women had improved sexual functioning and 9 men and 5 women had worse sexual functioning with a renal transplant as compared to hemodialysis. The remainder either said that they had no change, were not sure of the direction of change or did not answer this question [28]. In another study by *Salvatierra*, the sexual functioning of 130 male transplant patients was determined by questionnaire. Their data essentially replicated this study, but tended to show somewhat better sexual functioning of these patients [29].

As to the cause of the sexual dysfunction of these patients, much remains to be understood concerning the endocrinology of kidney failure. There have been some recent advances made in our knowledge of the sexual dysfunction of hemodialysis patients which point in the direction of organic factors playing a far more significant role than psychological ones [30, 31]. Since patients with renal transplantation often suffer from some degree of renal failure, that which is known about renal failure is at least partially applicable to the transplant group. Endocrine changes in kidney failure for men include: a decrease in testosterone levels, an increase in leutinizing hormone, and a diminution in testicular size and quantity of sperm. Women on dialysis tend to have cessation of menses. However, after transplantation menses often returns. Patients with a kidney transplantation who are on antihypertensive medication may experience a diminution in libido and of sexual ability as a side effect of their medication.

Concerning the psychological reasons for sexual dysfunction, many patients experience depression, in part due to the use of steroids. Among the somatic changes seen in depression are diminished sexual interest and ability. In addition, anxiety and depression may result because of either the precariousness patients experience about the possibility of rejection or else the actuality of kidney rejection. Sexual functioning is often an outlet in which difficulties in other areas of life are expressed. Emotional difficulties in transplant patients, irrespective of cause, may be reflected in problems of sexual functioning. It is therefore important that the transplant team be aware of the sexual problems of their patients so that they may be identified and appropriate treatment given. (Penile prostheses are discussed on p. 212.)

Treatment Considerations

Much of what we know about the psychological stresses of renal transplantation can be translated into treatment considerations [32–34]. From the preventative standpoint, the behaviorally trained physician, nurse and other health care professional can and should be of assistance to the transplant team in patient selection. Generally, very independent patients tend to do much better with transplantation than with dialysis. However, those with depression, or a strong propensity for depressive or psychotic disorders, tend not to do well with transplantation because of the need for postoperative steroids. Thus, transplantation should not be performed on such patients if another form of treatment for kidney failure is feasible.

Assistance should be given to the transplant team in the selection of live, related donors. Those potential donors with major ambivalence about the procedure or about the recipient should not be encouraged to donate their kidneys. Donors need to be educated concerning the practical considerations of their gift-giving. They need to know that the transplantation of their kidney will not result in the recipient being the same as he/she was prior to kidney failure. The best that can be expected is that rejection will be warded off under careful monitoring by the transplant team; that near normal life activities can be assumed without dependence upon dialysis. Nonetheless, there remains the possibility of the complications of long term steroid therapy.

The transplant team may need help in communicating to potential recipients the details about the operative procedure. Transplant surgeons should be encouraged to be clear, concise, and open in telling patients about the statistics of success and failure of the procedure, the details of post-operative morbidity and the complications of steroid therapy. Post-operatively, donors often need support in their feeling of being left out and now being off center stage. Renal recipients need careful monitoring as to psychosis and depression during their immunosuppressive treatment.

Last but not least, the liaison psychiatrist or other behaviorally trained professional working with transplant teams should consider staff education a primary goal of their work. This includes attending to the needs of the staff themselves by permitting its members to express their feelings about the difficult work that they do and for the staff to present the psychological problems of their patients to a person who may help them understand and respond constructively to it [35].

References

1   Salvatierra, O. Jr.; Amend, W.; Vicenti, F.: Pretreatment with donor-specific blood transfusions in related recipients with high MLC. Transplant. Proc. *13:* 142–149 (1981).
2   Luke, R.G.: Renal replacement therapy. N. Engl. J. Med. *308:* 1593–1595 (1983).
3   Krakauer, H.; Grauman, J.S.; McMullan, J.R.; Creede, C.C.: The recent U.S. experience in the treatment of end-stage renal disease by dialysis and transplantation. N. Engl. J. Med. *308:* 1558–1563 (1983).
4   Kemph, J.P.: Renal failure, artificial kidney and kidney transplant. Am. J. Psychiat. *122:* 1270–1274 (1966).
5   Cramond, W.A.; Knight, P.R.; Lawrence, J.R.: The psychiatric contribution to a renal unit undertaking chronic hemodialysis and renal homotransplantation. Br. J. Psychiat. *113:* 1201–1212 (1967).
6   Eisendrath, R.M.: The role of grief and fear in the death of kidney transplant patients. Am. J. Psychiat. *126:* 381–387 (1967).
7   Kemph, J.P.: Psychotherapy with patients receiving kidney transplant. Am. J. Psychiat. *124:* 623–629 (1967).

8   Crammond, W.A.: Renal homotransplantation; some observations on recipients and do-
     nors. Brit. J. Psychiat. *113:* 1223–1230 (1967).

9   Fellner, C.H.; Marshall, J.R.: Twelve kidney donors. J. Am. Med. Ass. *206:* 2703–2707
     (1968).

10   Ferris, G.N.: Psychiatric considerations in patients receiving cadaveric renal transplants.
     Soc. Med. J. *62:* 1482–1484 (1969).

11   Castelnuovo-Tedesco, P. (ed.): Psychiatric aspects of organ transplantation. (Grune and
     Stratton, New York 1971).

12   Muslin, H.L.: On acquiring a kidney. Am. J. Psychiat. *127:* 1185–1188 (1971).

13   Abram, H.S.: Psychological dilemmas of medical progress. Psychiat. in Med. *3:* 51–57
     (1972).

14   Castelnuovo-Tedesco, P.: Organ transplant, body image psychosis. Psychoanal. Quart. *42:*
     344–363 (1973).

15   Basch, S.H.: The intrapsychic integration of a new organ: a clinical study of kidney
     transplantation. Psychoanal. Quart. *42:* 364–384 (1973).

16   Viederman, M.: The search for meaning in renal transplantation. Psychiat. *37:* 283–290
     (1974).

17   Fox, R.C.; Swazey, J.P.: The courage to fail: a social view of organ transplants and dialysis.
     (University of Chicago Press, Chicago 1974).

18   Simmons, R.G.: Psychological reactions to giving a kidney; in Levy, Psychonephrology 1:
     psychological factors in hemodialysis & transplantation; pp. 227–245 (Plenum, New York
     1983).

19   Beard, B.: The quality of life before and after renal transplantation. Dis. Nerv. System.
     32: 24–31 (1971).

20   Abram, H.S.: The psychiatrist and the treatment of chronic renal failure and the prolonga-
     tion of life. Am. J. Psychiat. *128:* 1534–1539 (1972).

21   George, J.: Life with a transplanted kidney. Med. J. Austral. *10:* 461 (1970).

22   Hamburg, D.; Adams, J.: A perspective on coping behavior. Arch. Gen. Psychiat. *17:*
     277–284 (1967).

23   Crombez, J.C.; Lefebvre, P.: The behavioral responses of renal transplant patients as seen
     through their fantasy life. Can. Psychiat. Assoc. J. *17* (Suppl. 2: 55): 19–72 (1972).

24   Steinberg, J.; Levy, N.B.; Radvila, A.: Psychological factors affecting acceptance or rejec-
     tion of kidney transplants; in Levy, Psychonephrology 1: psychological factors in
     hemodialysis and transplantation; pp. 185–217 (Plenum, New York 1981).

25   Fellner, C.J.: Selection of living kidney donors and the problem of informed consent; in
     Castelnuovo-Tedesco, ed., Psychiatric aspects of organ transplantation; pp. 79–85 (Grune
     & Stratton, New York 1971).

26   Simmons, R.G.; Klein, S.D.; Simmons, R.L.: Gift of life: the social and psychological
     impact of organ transplantation. (Wiley Interscience, New York 1977).

27   Haynes, R.C.; Murad, F.: Adrenocorticotropic hormone; in Gilman; Goodman and Gil-
     man's the pharmacological basis of therapeutics; p. 1483 (Macmillan, New York 1980).

28   Levy, N.B.: Sexual adjustment to maintenance hemodialysis and renal transplantation:
     national survey by questionnaire: preliminary report. Trans. Am. Soc. Artif. Int. Organs.
     19: 138–142 (1973).

29   Salvatierra, O.; Fortmann, J.L.; Belzer, F.O.: Sexual function in males before and after
     transplantation. Urol. *5:* 64 (1975).

30   Procci, W.R.; Goldstein, D.A.; Kletzky, O.A.; Campese, V.M.; Massry, S.G.: Impotence

in uremia: preliminary results of a combined medical and psychiatric investigation; in Levy, Psychonephrology 2: psychological problems in kidney failure and their treatment; pp. 235–246 (Plenum, New York 1983).

31   Procci, W.R.; Goldstein, D.A.; Adelstein, J.: Sexual dysfunction in the male uremic patient: a reappraisal. Kid. Internat. *19:* 317–323 (1982).

32   Freyberger, H.: The renal transplant patients: three-stage model and psychotherapeutic strategies; in Levy, Psychonephrology 2: psychological problems in kidney failure and their treatment; pp. 259–265 (Plenum, New York 1983).

33   Burley, J.: A model for social work intervention in live-related kidney transplantation; in Levy, Psychonephrology 2: psychological problems in kidney failure and their treatment; pp. 267–274 (Plenum, New York 1983).

34   Simmons, R.G.: Long-term reactions of renal recipients and donors; in Levy, Psychonephrology 2: psychological problems in kidney failure and their treatment; pp. 275–287 (Plenum, New York 1983).

35   Levy, N.: Psychological complications of dialysis: Psychonephrology to the rescue. Bull. Menn. Clin. *48:* 237–250 (1984).

Norman B. Levy, MD, Westchester County Medical Center, Valhalla, NY 10595 (USA)

Adv. psychosom. Med., vol. 15, pp. 180–198 (Karger, Basel 1986)

Hysterectomy and Tubal Ligation

Maggie Ryan, Lorraine Dennerstein

Departments of Psychiatry and Obstetrics and Gynaecology, University of Melbourne, Melbourne, Australia

Gynaecological surgery poses a unique stress for women because of the identification of the reproductive organs both with sexuality and with the wider concept of feminine identity. This stress is particularly apparent when one considers that surgery, such as hysterectomy and tubal ligation, can produce loss of an important female role – the ability to bear a child. The indications and processes associated with both these gynaecological procedures differ vastly. The loss of fertility is usually voluntary in the case of tubal ligation but may be involuntary when hysterectomy is performed because of gynaecological disorder. The incidence of these procedures has increased rapidly over recent years, particularly in the Western world. It has been estimated that 50% of women in the USA will undergo hysterectomy operation in their lifetime [1]. For 60–65 million couples world wide, female sterilization is the chosen method of fertility control. In North America 6 million women have made this choice [2] and it is the most common method of birth control in the United States for women in the 30–44 age group [3].

The problems of mortality and physical morbidity in relation to these procedures have largely been solved but because these procedures affect the exclusive and important female role of child bearing, the questions now most frequently being asked, but which still remain inadequately answered, relate to the psychological sequelae. Findings from the many studies which address this issue are confusing and sometimes contradictory, usually due to methodological inadequacies in research design. However, as with surgical techniques, research techniques and methods of data analysis continue to improve. Some recent studies give promise of progress in our knowledge in these areas.

Methodological Problems

Early research tended to be retrospective in design. These studies suffer the basic flaw of 'one shot design', in that we cannot assume that any psychological disturbance found in patients after surgery was not present beforehand. The real value of such studies is in the questions raised for further research, for example, the vulnerability of certain categories of patients. Another feature of earlier studies was the lack of standardized measures to assess outcome. Clinical interviews have disadvantages in that, under these conditions observer bias may be allowed to operate. In addition, comparisons between studies are difficult, and consequently, knowledge in the area does not accumulate in any systematic fashion.

Sampling is another unsatisfactory aspect. Some samples are too small for meaningful analysis, others have high attrition rates, while still other samples mix patients that undergo a procedure for different reasons, e.g. patients who have chosen tubal ligation for a strictly medical reason are likely to have problems different from those who have chosen sterilization for contraception.

In the case of hysterectomy, study samples sometimes include women who undergo surgery for benign and malignant reasons. Some studies included patients who had undergone both hysterectomy and oophorectomy. It is not always clear whether hormone replacement therapy had been administered.

In an excellent review and analysis of the literature on contraceptive sterilization, *Schwyhart* [4] in 1973 pointed to the need for longitudinal study with standardized measures, involvement of couples rather than women only and a need to look at quality of life issues. This chapter focuses on recent research into some types of gynaecological surgery. Unfortunately, Schwyhart's timely reminder has escaped the notice of many researchers.

Tubal Ligation

Changing Attitudes Towards Sterilization

Until the late 1960s in England and Australia, the medical profession still had lingering doubts as to the legality of sterilization for reasons other than therapeutic. Thus, until that time, women having this surgery usually did so for medical reasons. We would expect the outcome for these women to be influenced by their pre-existing health conditions, and by the absence of choice which sometimes existed precisely because of the nature of an existing health condition. Whilst they would have consented to surgery, they may not have actively desired it, as would well-informed healthy women who consciously chose this as their preferred method of birth control. The values held in society today encourage and indeed, expect women to make responsible decisions about family planning. Therefore, the attitudes of the medical profession, which reflect these values, are more positive towards sterilization. This in itself is likely to affect outcome. As research shows, the situation in societies more traditional in outlook, and with less educated populations, may be entirely different. For this reason, when we review the literature in this whole area, we cannot help but be aware of the effects of evolving medical technology, research technology, and societal and cultural values.

Psychological Sequelae

Early studies of psychological sequelae of tubal ligation were reviewed critically by *Schwyhart* [4]. This report will focus on the more recent studies following the change in medical attitudes to sterilization.

The rate of psychiatric morbidity varied greatly from 60% [5] to a study that demonstrated no psychiatric sequelae attributable to this operation (*Sim* [6]). This contradictory situation is largely the result of the methodological problems already described. In general, retrospective studies suggest a higher rate of psychiatric sequelae. The study by *Enoch* et al. [5] found at follow-up that 60% of the sample had suffered a psychiatric illness following the surgery. The high rate becomes understandable when one notes that only 34% had requested the surgery; the remaining women were 'advised' (by their doctors) to accept sterilization because of parity, marital problems, medical and/or psychiatric reasons. Those women who underwent surgery for the reason of high parity were more likely to have successful outcomes than those for whom other reasons were indicated. Another possible source of bias in this study is the diminished sample. One third of the women invited to participate did not do so. Another study which found a high incidence of psychiatric sequelae reported that 51% of the sample of 49 considered their mental state to have deteriorated when they were interviewed 6 months after surgery [7]. In this study one of the outcome parameters was the consumption of alcohol. 14% of the women reported increased alcohol intake at follow-up. Again, this was a mixed sample and those patients for whom high parity was the major reason for undergoing surgery had a better result. Personality factors were also found to effect outcome. In contrast, *Sims* et al. [6] in a retrospective study using a structured questionnaire, found no psychiatric sequelae that could be attributed to the surgery.

Of the prospective studies, the following three report high rates of adverse psychological sequelae [8, 9, 10]. None utilized standardized measures of outcome. Instead outcome was determined by psychiatric interview or patient self report. The *Indian study* [8] found 83% of patients to be describing psychological symptoms when reviewed 3–24 months following surgery but these were mild in nature and the authors report symptoms such as depression and anxiety to be absent. The high incidence of physical symptoms may possibly reflect the role cultural factors play in symptom formation. The Belgian study of *Cliquet* et al. [10] reported 22% of the sample seen at 4 months follow-up indicated negative psychological reactions, such as depression, anxiety and guilt feelings. The authors attributed these reactions to incomplete physical recovery at that stage and insufficient support from partners. A reduced sample of patients was seen by the authors at 12 months follow-up. Unfortunately there was no further report on the psychological aspects of the study. The Chicago study by *Campanella and Wolfe* [9] of a sample which reviewed patients at 6 months, 1 year and 2 years following surgery, found younger patients, i.e. those less than 26 years, more likely to have complaints.

The more recent prospective studies by *Smith* [11] and *Cooper* et al. [12] have the advantage of better methodology. Both arrived at conclusions quite different from the studies described above. In her Scottish study, Smith [11] used Goldberg's General Health Questionnaire and a standardized psychiatric interview to define psychiatric outcome for 196 consecutively referred women. At the initial pre-operative assessment, 25% of the women had scores of 12 or more, a significantly higher rate than found in the general population [13]. Following sterilization these scores improved so that only 4.5% had scores of 12 or more at 12 months follow-up interview when the attrition rate was 15%. In their prospective study of women who had interval sterilization *Cooper* et al. [12] interviewed women 4 weeks before, plus 6 and 18 months after tubal ligation. Attrition rate was only 5.5%. The measure used for psychological outcome was the Present State Examination of *Wing* [14]. The prevalence of psychiatric morbidity beforehand was 10.4% which is no more than might be expected in the population. This was reduced to 4.7% at the 6 months interview and was 9.3% at the 12 months post-operative follow-up interview. Only 12 people who were not 'cases' (as defined by the level of the PSE score) developed psychiatric symptoms at 18 months.

Conversely, 15 of the 21 'cases' beforehand had improved to become 'non-cases'.

Sexual Adjustment

Again, the approach differs from study to study with the recent prospective studies giving a more optimistic picture. Of the retrospective studies, *Ansare and Francis* [7] found that 78% of patients reported either no change or an improvement in their sexual lives. Of the remainder, 22% reported that this aspect of their lives was negatively affected by the surgery. *Enoch and Jones* [5] found 44% to have improved sexual relations, but 22% complained of loss of libido. 51% of those replying to *Jackson's* [15] questionnaire in New Zealand reported their sexual life unchanged and 18% reported 'loss of libido'. *Cooper* et al. [12] in his prospective study, used a more objective measure of sexual adjustment. Patients were asked to report on frequency and enjoyment. 18 months after surgery, 28% of patients were reporting increased frequency, 26% decreased frequency, and for 46% this aspect remained unchanged. However, when rating enjoyment, only 3.2% reported that sexual intercourse was less enjoyable since surgery. *Smith* [11], in her prospective study, asked patients to rate sexual satisfaction on four points from very satisfactory to unsatisfactory. For 34% of the sample, satisfaction was better; 8% worse, and 58% reported no change. *Campanella and Wolfe's* [9] figures were presented more obscurely. However, it would appear that the numbers who found sexual satisfaction diminished were small, but the younger women, i.e. those under 26 years of age, were more likely than the older women to be adversely affected.

Dissatisfaction, Regret and Request for Reversal

Regret is a more difficult area to research as even standardized measures may not give an accurate reflection of the patients' feelings. Estimates of regret vary. *Schwyhart* [3] estimated regret occurred in between one to 18%. *Cooper* [12] reported 10.9% experienced regret, but only 3.1% would have considered reversal. Some women may regret the operation but on a rational basis acknowledge its necessity on realistic grounds such as a medical condition which precludes other forms of contraception. Such women may report experiencing regret but would nevertheless take the same course of action again and do not consider reversal. For others regret may follow because the initial decision was hasty or uninformed or the situation which made sterilization seem desirable, e.g. a poor marital relationship or economic circumstances may have changed. These women may then regret the earlier decision and may seek reversal.

For these reasons, study findings relating to dissatisfaction or regret are not particularly helpful unless they also specify reasons for regret. *Winston* [16] studied the reasons for 103 women requesting reversal at Hammersmith Hospital. He noted that more than would have been expected were sterilized at a young age (the mean age at sterilization for this group was 26.7 years) and more than half had been sterilized immediately after delivery or abortion. These patients usually gave several reasons for being sterilized but it is interesting to note that 75.7% had reported their marriages to be so unhappy at the time that they felt they could not cope with more children. 78% of those requesting reversal were doing so because they had remarried or had formed new relationships. Some requested reversal in the hope of improving their sexual relationships. Recent developments in amniocentesis prompted 4 patients who had been sterilized for genetic reasons to seek reversal. Another English Study by *Thompson and Templeton* [17] gives a similar picture. These authors emphasized the necessity for adequate counseling prior to sterilization.

Factors Associated with Vulnerability

Although there is some disagreement, certain themes emerge from the literature which indicate to the clinician those women who may be at risk for adverse sequelae and who, therefore, need more careful counseling before they reach a final decision about terminating fertility. These factors will be reviewed.

Age

It has been suggested that young women are at more risk for an adverse reaction to tubal ligation [6, 16]; however, other findings are in contrast [5, 12, 18].

Marital Problems

Several studies indicate that patients who experience adverse sequelae following sterilization, express regret or requested reversal had also been experiencing marital disharmony at the time of the decision to have sterilization [11, 12, 16, 18]. Several others recommend that patients who are experiencing marital problems at the time of their request for sterilization should receive counseling in relation to that problem, as concerns about fertility are likely to be only one aspect of the factors involved in such relationships. In these cases, changing circumstances such as separation, reconciliation, or a new marriage may alter the patient's view of sterilization. It is interesting to note that the majority of patients in Winston's study asking for reversal had new partners at the time of their request.

Parity

Early studies frequently cited low parity as a risk factor. However, recent studies do not support this [11, 12], perhaps reflecting changing community attitudes to family size. In a follow-up of 45 nulliparous women who had undergone tubal ligations, *Benjamin* et al. [19] found that 11.4% of the women expressed unhappiness about their operation; but for most of these women the surgery was performed for medical reasons.

Previous Psychiatric History and Personality Factors

Some studies report association between pre-operative psychiatric history and adverse outcome [5, 12]. Others do not [6, 11]. Personality variables were found to associate with outcome in other studies [5, 7, 9].

Timing of Surgery

The consensus of studies is clearly that there are less undesirable sequelae when women undergo interval sterilization rather than when the operation is performed at the time of abortion or caesarean section [6].

Pathways to Surgery

This area has received little attention but some authors note that those patients who requested sterilization themselves had better outcomes than those patients who had been 'persuaded' or to whom this course had been 'suggested' [6, 7]. *Campanella* [9] suggests that those patients who were not well informed about the procedure and its outcome risk a poor result.

Clinical Implications

Whilst being inconclusive, the literature provides sufficient indication to the clinician that the decision to choose tubal ligation as the means of fertility control should only be taken by patients who are well informed as to its effect and outcome. The decision should be an informed one of the couple after both have been adequately counseled about contraceptive alternatives; it should not be taken in haste. Special care should be taken with young patients or those who have marital problems, sexual difficulties, neurotic personalities or who have unrealistic ideas of what this surgery may achieve for them in their personal lives.

There are a number of ways in which psychiatrists may become involved with patients who undergo tubal ligation. Initially they may be asked to assess a woman's or couple's suitability for the procedure. In doing so, the psychiatrist will assess the couple's knowledge about, and expectations of, contraceptive methods including sterilization. The couple's age, personalities, previous psychiatric morbidity, parity, sexual and general relationship will also be evaluated bearing in mind the risk factors for regret of the operation. Sometimes it may be the psychiatrist who recommends to a patient that she should be sterilized. This may be related to the risk of psychiatric or other illness following childbirth: for example, a woman who has already suffered 2 episodes of post-partum psychosis. Alternatively, the psychiatrist may be referred a patient because of psychiatric or sexual maladjustment following tubal ligation. Patients presenting with such problems need full evaluation. Women who have lost interest in sex following the loss of childbearing may be helped by a combination of psychotherapeutic and sex therapy statagems.

Hysterectomy

Hysterectomy has long been reputed to be followed by a high incidence of psychological and sexual sequelae. One of the earliest reports of adverse outcome [20] was that made by a Venetian professor, *Giacomo Berengario da Carp* (1480–1550), who recorded that his father had removed the gangrenous uterus of a patient. She lived for many years afterwards, resumed sexual relations with her husband, but experienced little sexual satisfaction. Towards the end of the 19th century, *Von Krafft-Ebing* [21] observed that psychosis followed hysterectomy more frequently than it did other surgical procedures. Half a century passed and countless hysterectomies were performed before this issue was again taken up by *Lindemann* [22].

Early writers such as *Deutsch* [23] and *Drellick and Bieber* [24] emphasized loss of child bearing capacity in terms of women's feminine self-concepts. These studies also focused on the symbolic significance of the uterus, both the conscious and unconscious perceptions of uterine value and use, and women's expectations of the effects of surgery. More recently the crisis nature of hysterectomy has been emphasized and the process of adaptation to stresses involved explored [25, 26].

Of particular interest was a study demonstrating the prolonged and phasic nature of the pattern of adaptation [27], reporting firstly a blocking out or avoidance of the realization of the traumatic event (denial) with later gradual admittance to consciousness. In this manner the trauma is gradually accepted, with its accompanying discomfort. If the trauma is not worked through in this manner, the patient may become symptomatic in a fashion described as the Stress Response Syndrome [27].

There are 3 questions of interest to clinicians in terms of coping with gynaecological surgery. The first relates to the frequency of hysterectomy. Why is there such a high frequency of hysterectomy in the Western world, such that nearly every second woman in the USA and Australia will have her uterus removed by the age of 65? [1] Why does the frequency vary in different countries – is there less pathology in Britain where the rate of hysterectomy is half that of the USA?

The second question relates to the sequelae of this surgery: what are the types and incidence of psychological and sexual sequelae: and who are at risk?

The third question relates to management – what sort of interventions pre-operatively and post-operatively from the family doctor or gynaecologist are likely to lead to less sequelae and to help the woman cope more effectively with surgery? What can be done to help the woman after surgery?

Frequency of Hysterectomy

Whilst it is difficult to obtain exact figures, it would appear that there is an astonishingly high frequency of hysterectomy in many countries. Indeed it is so high that in countries such as the USA and Australia, women are now being encouraged by health insurance funds to seek a second opinion before agreeing to hysterectomy. Although hysterectomy may be performed for organic causes, still in many women there is no demonstrable pathology. Possible reasons include functional, menstruation related complaints. It may be that an increase in these complaints is related to an increase in smoking and drinking alcohol, as these habits are associated with increased menstrual complaints. It is also possible that women in the Western world may now perceive as abnormal, menstrual blood loss and/or discomfort which would previously have been tolerated. A possible reason for this lowered tolerance of menstruation may have been the long term use of the oral contraceptive pill which usually produces a marked reduction in the amount of bleeding and discomfort experienced. Women are often advised to cease the 'Pill' after the age of 35 and use other forms of contraception. Some women then find the return to 'normal' menstruation intolerable.

A major concern is that when women complain of heavy periods this does not necessarily mean heavy blood loss. Prolonged heavy blood loss would lead to anemia and ill-health; hysterectomy is indeed justifiable to prevent this. When women who complain of heavy periods were studied, only 50% had evidence of increased blood loss and only a much smaller percentage were anemic [28]. Blood may comprise only 20% of the total fluid content of menstruation and yet it is this component that is so important in determining therapy. The number of sanitary pads or tampons used bears little or no relationship to the actual amount of blood loss.

Other factors also influence the amount of blood loss. For example, in many primitive societies menstrual flow is scanty and usually only lasts one day. Nutrition may be an important factor. It is important to reflect that regular menstruation is an artifact of modern society. In more primitive societies, the menarche or first period occurred later, the menopause earlier and pregnancy and prolonged breast feeding (with associated lack of periods) occupied much of the interim period.

In an evolutionary sense we have not had time for our bodies to adjust to the tremendous changes wrought by our modern contraceptive technology. This may be a major reason for women in Western countries expressing dissatisfaction with their periods and seeking hysterectomy. There are now available medications which help reduce the amount of bleeding and pain. These may not be acceptable to all patients or be completely successful in eradicating symptoms.

Another major factor which may influence both the amount of menstrual blood loss, plus the discomfort, tolerance, and perception of this, is the emotional state. Studies in the U.K. [29], USA [30] and Australia [31] have found an extraordinarily high number of women (55%, 57% and 47%) to be suffering from significant emotional illness pre-hysterectomy. The incidence of such symptoms in the general population is only 12–14%. The main types of psychiatric problems suffered were those of depression and anxiety.

How can we interpret these findings? It is possible that at least some of these psychological problems represented anxiety about the forthcoming operation. In the U.K. study [29] women may have been waiting to have the operation for some time. When it is known that the operation is needed, a long wait may have increased anxiety. Interestingly, over half of the patients with psychiatric problems had significantly improved when interviewed 18 months post-operatively [32].

Another major explanation of the presence pre-operatively of such a large number of women with psychiatric problems is that women with psychological problems or some inner distress may present to doctors with gynaecological symptoms. In our society negative attitudes to mental illness are common. Women with psychological distress may tend to present to their doctors saying 'I feel sick' rather than 'I feel sad or miserable or nervous'. Our whole medical system seems to encourage this focus on physical complaints rather than emotional. As one of our patients remarked after hysterectomy, 'I go to the doctor when I feel bad, but I always seem to get the wrong thing', by which she meant operations, instead of treatment for her emotional problems. It is well known that when people do feel depressed or anxious, they often focus on bodily symptoms and tend to perceive these more negatively.

Lastly, it is possible that psychiatric problems may adversely influence the menstrual cycle.

Gynaecologists obviously have a major influence in the rate of hysterectomy, as they must make the final recommendation that such an operation is necessary. In making a diagnosis, the gynaecologist relies on the description of the illness provided by the patient, and examination of the patient. Yet as already described, it may be unrealistic to expect women to be accurate reporters of such symptoms as blood loss. The distribution and availability of gynaecological surgeons in a population may also be an important determinant of the operative rate. There are more gynaecologists per head of population in both Australia and North America than the United Kingdom which has a lower hysterectomy rate. There is no doubt that some doctors and some patients are more surgically oriented, whilst others are more drug oriented. Some women have the operation as an alternative to sterilization, particularly if they wish to stop menstruation.

It is obviously important for the clinician to be aware of the factors which may be influencing the pathway to hysterectomy in making a decision about whether hysterectomy is indicated for an individual woman.

Incidence of Psychological and Sexual Sequelae after Hysterectomy

Many retrospective studies test the hypothesis that, because of the symbolic significance of the uterus, hysterectomy is followed by a higher incidence of psychological and sexual disorders. Several authors found evidence of adverse psychological or sexual sequelae: i.e. an increased psychiatric-hospital admission rate compared with other surgery or with expected community rates [33] (the most frequent diagnosis was depression); an increased incidence of psychiatric referral [34] (especially for depression); an increased frequency of treatment with antidepressants in a general-practitioner setting [35, 36]; and deterioration of the sexual relationship of many patients after hysterectomy [35, 37].

Meikle et al. [38] quoted 8 studies which failed to find adverse consequences of hysterectomy. In 3 of these studies there was an increased incidence of adverse sequelae. *Munday and Cox* [39] reported that 33⅓% of their sample reported emotional distress. *Bragg* [40] found the risk for psychiatric-hospital admission to be slightly greater after hysterectomy than after cholecystectomy, although the difference was not statistically significant. *Patterson and Craig* (41) studied 100 female psychiatric inpatients who had undergone hysterectomy. Because only 15% were admitted in the first year after hysterectomy, these authors concluded that the hysterectomy itself was not a particularly stressful experience. The other studies cited by *Meikle* suffered from methodological difficulties, including failure to report the method or measures used [42, 43] and high attrition rates [44]. One author [45] reported that he 'interrogated' his patients.

Retrospective studies cannot yield conclusive evidence as to whether there are adverse sequelae of hysterectomy, because they cannot provide us with information about the patient's psychological and sexual well-being before the operation. Prospective design is needed to provide conclusive evidence of the effects of hysterectomy.

Early prospective studies were mainly exploratory and descriptive, with little quantitative data or statistical analysis in the reports. *Lindemann* [22, 24] did include a control group and a careful examination of past and current psychiatric status, but he failed to indicate how many of his small sample had undergone hysterectomy. These studies [22, 24] did, however, identify risk factors for poor outcome.

Barglow [46] compared the outcome after hysterectomy with that after tubal ligation. Since the women studied had neither actively sought sterilization nor had a choice of surgical procedure, it is hardly surprising that there was a worse outcome for the more final operation of hysterectomy. *Chynoweth* [47] and *Raphael* [26] investigated the general health outcome and sexual response after hysterectomy. Both reports suffer from brevity, which makes it difficult to follow the method used. Apparently, the same tests were not applied pre- and post-operatively, and therefore the evaluation of health impairment became rather subjective, with little more validity than that reached by retrospective studies. Furthermore, although both chief investigators were psychiatrists, no mention is made of the psychiatric health of patients pre-operatively.

In 3 studies [38, 48, 49], no significant change in the parameters studied was found after hysterectomy. The same measures were used pre- and post-operatively, but the duration of follow-up was probably too short (3–6 months) in view of the many studies which suggest that the process of adjustment to hysterectomy may take 12–24 months. One of these studies [46] had a 42% drop-out rate, probably reflecting the technique of leaving rating scales with the patients for completion and return.

The recent studies done by *Martin* et al. [30, 50] and *Gath* [29, 32] are of considerable interest. Both utilized intensive psychiatric interviews and psychological rating scales both pre- and post-operatively. There are some interesting similarities and differences between these studies. Different criteria for psychiatric illness were used and different rating scales. The investigators also differed: in one case a male psychiatrist in a hospital setting [30, 50] and in the other female social workers and psychologists who visited the patients in their own homes [29, 32].

Prior to the operation, both study populations had extremely similar incidences of psychiatric illness (55–57%). The type of diagnosis varied. This may reflect real differences in the women studied or their pathways to surgery. For example, the British women had to wait for surgery and may have been understandably more anxious by the time of operation. Since the hysterectomy rate in the USA is twice that of the U.K., it is possible that more women with Briquet's syndrome are operated on in the USA. Alternatively, the difference in type of diagnosis might simply reflect the different criteria used. The Present State Examination used by *Gath* has no separate category recognising Briquet's syndrome. In a recent prospective study by the present authors [31] a high rate of psychiatric morbidity pre-operatively was also found. This study investigated 30 women prior to hysterectomy using the Present State Examination as a measure of psychological health and also sought to identify Briquet's syndrome using *Feighner's* criteria. Only one woman in the sample received this diagnosis, in contrast to 27% in the *Martin* et al. study.

These recent prospective studies raise some interesting hypotheses. It would seem that the incidence of development of new psychiatric problems is small and that most psychiatric problems will occur in those who had psychiatric problems pre-operatively. It is interesting to speculate whether this has always been the case or is perhaps a reflection of the tremendous social changes of the past few decades: the de-emphasis of reproduction for women's self-esteem and the increase in women's knowledge about their bodies as well as their more active participation in their interaction with doctors. The 2 recent British studies [32, 51] further suggest that the support provided by trial interviews may even have decreased the psychiatric morbidity in patients. This has obvious implications for the prevention of psychological sequelae.

Clinical Implications

How can the clinician lessen the likelihood of sequelae and help women successfully adapt to surgery? (For further information on this subject, refer to p. 23, 'Psychological intervention with surgical patients evaluation outcome'.)

Pre-Operative Management

Psychological preparation should be carried out routinely in the same way as the patient is prepared for the physical aspects of the operation. Extra time or care may be needed with patients identified as being at risk of a poor outcome. The major risk factor for a poor outcome after hysterectomy is the presence of psychiatric morbidity before the operation as revealed by interview, personality rating scales and a history of previous referal to a psychiatrist [32, 50]. A summary of risk factors identified elsewhere in the literature suggests that other risk factors for a poor outcome after hysterectomy will include: younger age [26]; lower educational status [47]; absence of any concern pre-operatively or excessive anxiety [52]; absence of perceived support in the immediate social network [26]; poor relationship with mother [47]; and negative expectations of the operation [37].

The purpose of pre-operative preparation is to lessen anxiety about the possible effects of the surgery. This is best achieved in a supportive, empathic relationship where the patient is encouraged to discuss her feelings about the operation, and to relate what she may have heard from others about the effects of hysterectomy. An educative approach by the doctor will help dispel anxiety based on inadequate knowledge. Information on the anatomy and physiology of the reproductive system and genital organs in simple language, with the aid of diagrams, is helpful to most patients. The nature of the operation, the reasons for it, and the expected changes can then be elaborated. Advice should be given on when normal activities, particularly sexual intercourse, may be resumed. As anxiety may limit the recall of information, this explanation may need to be repeated on several occasions or reinforced with a book suitable for women to read at home, such as 'Hysterectomy: How to deal with the Physical and Emotional Aspects' [53]. Where applicable, and if the partner is willing, it is desirable that he should be included in order to allay possible anxiety about the likely effects of hysterectomy and help him to understand the type of support his partner needs. Encouragement to discuss the operation is usually extremely beneficial. Ideally this should occur pre-operatively or, if this is not practical, in the immediate post-operative period.

The value of pre-operative preparation was shown in an Israeli study which explored further the findings of *Dennerstein* et al. [37] of an association between negative expectations of hysterectomy and deterioration of sexual function. Women in the hospital undergoing hysterectomy were randomly assigned to a two hour group discussion on hysterectomy or to the usual preparation by their gynaecologist. The women who had attended the single group sessions were later found to be significantly better adjusted psychologically and sexually [54]. This study demonstrates how even minimum intervention or one session spent discussing the operation can have marked benefits for the patient.

Hormone Therapy

Coppen et al. [51] have demonstrated that oestrogen therapy was of no benefit to premenopausal hysterectomised women with intact ovaries. Following bilateral oophorectomy or menopause, however, prophylactic hormone replacement therapy is indicated. In such patients oestrogen administration will alleviate hot flushes, associated insomnia and fatigue and prevent dyspareunia due to atrophic vaginal changes. We have also found a beneficial effect of oestrogen on mood and parameters of sexual response such as sexual desire, enjoyment, vaginal lubrication and orgasmic frequency in our studies of oophorectomized women [55, 56].

Other long term benefits of oestrogen replacement must also be considered such as the prevention of osteoporosis. Against the benefits of oestrogen therapy must balance the risks, such as those of thrombo-embolism and exacerbation of diabetes or uterine cancer.

Follow-Up

Therapeutic effects of follow-up interviews were suggested by the study of *Coppen* et al. [51]. Long term follow-up by the family doctor or gynaecologist will help facilitate adaptation to hysterectomy. This follow-up should continue for 12 months as many problems may only become evident some months following surgery.

Therapy for Post-Hysterectomy Depression

Psychiatric disorders occurring after hysterectomy should be evaluated and managed initially in the same way as disorders presenting at other times of life. A woman referred, suffering from depression some months after hysterectomy should have a full psychiatric, mental state and physical examination performed.

The severity of the depression should be assessed and treatment of the depression begun accordingly. Any woman who is a suicide risk should be admitted to hospital. Those with moderate or severe depression are usually commenced on antidepressants. Where the depression is so severe as to be life threatening or there has been no response to antidepressants, electro-convulsive therapy may be used. Hormone replacement therapy for those who have symptoms of hormone deficiency or have undergone bilateral oophorectomy may also be indicated. As the depression begins to improve, the clinician can begin to explore gently the significance of the operation to the patient. It is also important to evaluate the reactions of others significant in the patient's life. Usually only supportive psychotherapy in combination with antidepressant medication is needed. Occasionally, a more intensive psychodynamically oriented psychotherapy is needed when the operation has triggered severe conflicts in the patient.

In summary, what is evident from the accumulated research is that there is a great deal of psychiatric disturbance present before hysterectomy. Whilst most psychiatric and sexual problems after hysterectomy occurred in those with pre-existing problems, some new cases also develop. Trial interviews may, in themselves, have been therapeutic for many women. The clinician has an important role to play – firstly in determining whether hysterectomy is indeed the correct therapy and what the woman's emotional as well as physical response is likely to be; secondly, in adequately preparing a woman and her partner for the operation – psychologically as well as physically; and, finally, in recognizing promptly those women who are having difficulty adapting to the operation and arranging prompt psychotherapeutic intervention.

References

1   Roeske, Nancy C.A.: Hysterectomy and the quality of life. Arch. Int. Med. *139:* 146–147 (1979).
2   Population Reports *8:* 5 C99–C122 (September 1980).
3   Westoff, C.F.: The modernization of U.S. contraceptive practice. Fam. Plan. Persp. *4:* 9–12 (1972).
4   Schwyhart, W.R.; Kutner, S.J.: A reanalysis of female reactions to contraceptive sterilization. J. Nerv. Ment. Dis. *156:* 354–370 (1973).
5   Enoch, D.M.; Jones, K.: Sterilization: A review of 98 sterilized women. Brit. J. Psychiat. *127:* 583–587 (1975).
6   Sim, M.; Emens, J.M.; Jordan, J.A.: Psychiatric aspects of female sterilization. Brit. Med. J. *3:* 220–223 (1973).
7   Ansari, J.M.A.; Francis, H.H.: A study of 49 sterilized females. Acta Psychiat. Scand. *54:* 315–322 (1976).
8   Khorana, A.B.; Vyas, A.A.: Psychological complications in women undergoing voluntary sterilization by salpingectomy. Brit. J. Psychiat. *127:* 67–71 (1975).
9   Campanella, R.; Wolff, J.R.: Emotional reaction to sterilization. Obs. Gyn. *45:* 331–334 (1975).
10 Cliquet, R.L.; Thiery, M.; Staelens, R.; Lambert, G.: J. Biosoc. Sci. *13:* 47–61 (1981).
11 Smith, Anne W.H.: Psychiatry aspects of sterilization: a prospective study. Brit. J. Psychiat. *135:* 304–309 (1979).
12 Cooper, C.; Gath, D.; Rose, N.; Fieldsend, R.: Psychological sequelae to elective sterilization: a prospective study. Brit. Med. J. *284:* 461–464 (1982).
13 Goldberg, D.P.; Kay, L.; Thompson, L.: Psychiatric morbidity in general practice and the community. Psychol. Med. *6:* 565–569 (1976).
14 Wing, J.K.; Cooper, J.E.; Sartorius, N.: Measurement and classification of psychiatric symptoms. Cambridge University Press 1974.
15 Jackson, P.: Female sterilization: a five year follow-up in Auckland. N. Z. Med. J. *91:* 140–143 (1980).

16 Winston, R.M.L.: Why 103 women asked for reversal of sterilization. Brit. Med. J. *2:* 305–307 (1980).

17 Thompson, P.; Templeton, A.: Characteristics of patients requesting reversal of sterilization. Brit. J. Obs. Gyn. *85:* 161–164 (1978).

18 Lawson, S.; Cole, R.A.; Templeton, A.A.: The effect of laparoscopic sterilization by diathermy or selastic bands on post-operative pain, menstrual symptoms and sexuality. Brit. J. Obs. Gyn. *86:* 659–663 (1979).

19 Benjamin, L.; Rubenstein, L.M.; Kleinkopf, V.: Elective sterilization in childless women. Fert. Steril. *34:* No. 2 (1980).

20 Ricci, V.: The genealogy of gynaecology: history of the development of gynaecology throughout the ages. (2000 BC–1800 AD), (The Blakiston Company, Philadelphia 1943).

21 Ackner, B.: Emotional aspects of hysterectomy: a follow-up of fifty patients under the age of 40. Adv. Psychosom. Med. *1:* 248 (1960).

22 Lindemann, E.: Observations on psychiatric sequelae to surgical operations in women. Am. J. Psychiat. *98:* 132 (1941).

23 Deutsch, H.: The psychology of women (Grune & Stratton, New York 1944).

24 Drellich, M.G.; Beiber, I.: The psychological importance of the uterus and its functions. J. Nerv. Disord. *126:* 322 (1958).

25 Raphael, B.: The crisis of hysterectomy. Aust. N. Z. J. Psychiat. *6:* 106 (1972).

26 Raphael, B.: Parameters of health outcome following hysterectomy. Am. J. Obstet. Gynecol. *118:* 417 (1974).

27 Kaltreider, N.B.; Wallace, A.; Horowitz, M.J.: A field study of the stress response syndrome. J. Am. Med. Assoc. *242:* 1499 (1979).

28 Fraser, I.: Perceptions of menstrual cycle symptomatology; in Dennerstein, L.; Burrows, G., (eds): Obstetrics gynaecology and psychiatry, pp. 97–104 (York Press, Melbourne 1981).

29 Gath, D.: Psychiatric aspects of hysterectomy; in Robins, L.; Clayton, P.; Wing, J. (eds): The social consequences of psychiatric illness (Brunner Mazel, Inc., New York 1980).

30 Martin, R.L.; Roberts, W.V.; Clayton, P.T.; Wetzel, R.: Psychiatric illness and non-cancer hysterectomy. Dis. Ner. Syst. *38:* 974–980 (1977).

31 Ryan, M.M.; Dennerstein, L.; Pepperell, R.T.: Preoperative psychological and sexual adjustment in hysterectomy patients; in Dennerstein, L.; Burrows, G. (eds): Obstetrics, gynaecology and psychiatry (York Press, Melbourne 1981).

32 Gath, D.; Cooper, P.; Day, A.: Hysterectomy and psychiatric disorder: Levels of psychiatric morbidity before and after hysterectomy. Brit. J. Psychiat. *140:* 335–350 (1982).

33 Hollender, M.C.: A study of patients admitted to a psychiatric hospital after pelvic operations. Amer. J. Obstet. Gynecol. *79:* 498 (1960).

34 Barker, M.G.: Psychiatric illness after hysterectomy. Brit. Med. J. *2:* 91 (1968).

35 Richards, D.H.: Depression after hysterectomy. Lancet *11:* 430 (1973).

36 Richards, D.H.: A post-hysterectomy syndrome. Lancet *11:* 983 (1974).

37 Dennerstein, L.; Wood, C.; Burrows, G.D.: Sexual response following hysterectomy and oophorectomy. Obstet. Gynecol. *49:* 92 (1977).

38 Meikle, S.; Brody, H.; Psych, F.: An investigation of the psychological effects of hysterectomy. J. Nerv. Ment. Dis. *164:* 36 (1979).

39 Munday, R.N.; Cox, L.W.: Hysterectomy for benign lesions. Med. J. Aust. *2:* 759 (1967).

40 Bragg, R.L.: Risk of admission to mental hospital following hysterectomy. Am. J. Publ.

Health *5:* 1403 (1965).

41 Patterson, R.M.; Craig, J.B.: Misconceptions concerning the psychological effects of hysterectomy. Am. J. Obstet. Gynecol. *85:* 104 (1963).

42 Hawkins, J.; Williams, D.: Total abdominal hysterectomy. J. Obstet. Gynaecol. Br. Commonw. *70:* 20 (1963).

43 Mills, W.G.: Depression after hysterectomy. Lancet *11:* 672 (1973).

44 Hampton, P.J.; Tarnasky, W.G.: Hysterectomy and tubal ligation. A comparison of the psychological aftermath. Am. J. Obstet. Gynecol. *119:* 949 (1974).

45 Huffman, J.W.: The effect of gynaecologic surgery on sexual relations. Am. J. Obstet. Gynecol. *59:* 915 (1950).

46 Barglow, P.: Pseudocyesis and psychiatric sequelae of sterilization. Arch. Gen. Psychiat. *2:* 571 (1964).

47 Chynoweth, R.: Psychological complication of hysterectomy. Aust. N.Z. J. Psychiat. *7:* 102 (1973).

48 Moore, J.T.; Tolley, D.H.: Depression following hysterectomy. Psychosomatics *17:* 86 (1976).

49 Richter, K.; Pieringer, W.; Mayer, H.G.K.: Psychological aspects of hysterectomy. Wien. Klin. Wschr. *88:* 733 (1976).

50 Martin, R.L.; Roberts, W.V.; Clayton, P.J.: Psychiatric status after hysterectomy. J. Am. Med. Ass. *244:* 350 (1980).

51 Coppen, A.; Bishop, M.; Beard, R.J.; et al.: Hysterectomy, hormones and behaviour. A prospective study. Lancet *1:* 126 (1981).

52 Menzer, D.; Morris, T.; Gates, P.; et al.: Patterns of emotional recovery from hysterectomy. Psychosom. Med. *5:* 379 (1957).

53 Dennerstein, L.; Wood, C.; Burrows, G.D.: Hysterectomy: How to deal with physical and emotional aspects (Oxford University, in press, Melbourne 1982).

54 Cohen, E.; Fela, L.; Gingold, A.; Goldman, J.: Paper presented at 3rd International Menopause Congress (Ostend 1981).

55 Dennerstein, L.; Burrows, G.D.; Hyman, G.; Wood, C.: Hormone therapy and affect. Maturitas *1:* 247 (1979).

56 Dennerstein, L.; Burrows, G.D.; Wood, C.; Hyman, G.: Hormones and sexuality: effect of oestrogen and progestogen. Obst. Gyn. *56:* 316–322 (1980).

Maggie Ryan, MD, Departments of Psychiatry and Obstetrics and Gynaecology, University of Melbourne, Parkville Victoria (Australia)

Adv. psychosom. Med., vol. 15, pp. 199–210 (Karger, Basel 1986)

Sequelae of Limb Amputation

Sherry G. Lundberg, Frederick G. Guggenheim

Instructor, Richland College, Dallas, Tex.; Chairman and Professor of Psychiatry, University of Arkansas for Medical Sciences, Little Rock, Ark., USA

Amputation of a body part dramatically alters physical reality and challenges the integrity of a person's subjective understanding of the self. While technology can provide a new amputee with sophisticated prosthetic devices which perform many functions as adequately as the original limb, re-establishing the individual's sense of self as a whole person psychologically and socially remains a formidable task.

The preponderance of clinical observations and experimental research indicates that early psychological evaluation and follow-up support therapies can have significant impact on both immediate post-surgical sequelae and long-term adjustment [1–3]. However, coordinated delivery of services that includes a psychological component is the exception rather than the rule [1, 3–7]. The psychiatrist in a hospital setting is a ideally placed to evaluate the patient pre- and post-surgery, to provide information and recommendations for the primary caregivers, and to give therapeutic support to the amputee. This chapter will examine issues of general adjustment with particular emphasis on the complex construct of body image as it relates to the loss of a body part.

Amputee Characteristics

The amputee population can be divided into 2 broad categories: disease-related amputees and traumatic amputees. Disease-induced amputation usually afflicts older persons who may be expected to have additional medical problems, while amputation resulting from a traumatic accident will more often be seen in younger, healthier individuals. Following the amputation, marked acute depression is generally not seen in diseased victims; rather, these individuals experience a chronic sense of helplessness, hopelessness and an inclination to become resigned to a totally disabled state. For these diseased amputees, themes of death are pervasive, and despair is evidenced by insomnia, anorexia, and withdrawal [8–10]. While a progressively deteriorating medical condition may allow time for the patient to accept the necessity of limb removal, many diseased amputees are confused by their ambivalence over the loss of a painful or useless body part [1]. The reality of a stump is hard to accept, and the vague optimism expressed before surgery dissolves rapidly under the stress of demanding rehabilitation tasks [2].

For the traumatic amputee, by contrast, the surgery may be over before the person realizes what has happened. In the absence of any time to prepare, the immediate post-operative response may be collapse of the usual coping mechanisms with some degree of personality disintegration [1]. Relief to be alive is frequently accompanied by denial of the consequences of the loss. Boastfulness and exhibitionistic behavior serve as masks for deep-seated anxieties [4, 11]. These amputees commonly express resentment and defiance rather than the hopelessness and despair of the diseased amputee. Anxieties are often focused on specific concerns related to job security, money and recreational opportunities [12]. The specific circumstances of the injury may preoccupy the traumatic victim during the first weeks post-amputation. Was something done dangerously wrong or foolishly heroic? Nightmares depicting the accident and its derivatives occur with themes centering on guilt and punishment, anger and blame.

Phases in the Post-Amputation Process

Acute and Sub-Acute Phase

In the acute phase, the major task of the amputee is to deal with the immediate reality of the operative intervention and its attendant circumstances. In the sub-acute phase, the patient deals with a variety of issues past, present and future, with the activities of daily life being of the greatest concern. In the chronic phase, the rehabilitation process winds down. For some, characteristically, there is acceptance and assimilation of the changed reality; for others, a continuing struggle with anger, frustration and sadness. Because amputees' approach the rehabilitation process from markedly divergent circumstances with regard to age, energy level, health status, psychodynamics and aspirations, there is no simple, neat time table of recovery nor sharp demarcation of phases.

Certain realities exist for all amputees. The normal body structure has been irreversibly altered and feelings of anxiety, shock, grief, anger, frustration, and self-pity occur predictably during the early weeks and months post-surgery. Reactions to seeing the stump for the first time may include feelings of deformity and revulsion, with a sense of deprivation resulting from experiencing the self as only part of a person [1].

Psychological responses to the amputation are highly individualistic. Some patients newly dealing with loss present as emotionally volatile, others appear isolated and even withdrawn. The newly altered state of the amputee creates a condition in which the gratification of a number of human needs, including those of love, acceptance and status, may be in jeopardy. In addition, activities which release energy and satisfy inner urges are thwarted. Emotional upset often peaks during the first week after amputation and later again at time of discharge [13]. It is during these periods that the amputee must face mastering activities of daily living while interacting with other people in new and different ways.

From the moment the patient awakes from amputation, there evolves a continuum of necessary psychological activities which include grieving for the lost part [13], maintaining self-esteem [1], reworking interpersonal relationships [14], and modifying personal and vocational values and goals [6]. The perceptual discrepancy between the present actual body and the body as reflected in the mind's eye must be reconciled [15].

Amputees typically experience considerable, though often masked, dysphoria throughout the rehabilitation process according to research studies [9, 16] and clinical observation [1, 11]. The *Caplan and Hackett* [9] study of aged lower limb amputees found that while depression was not readily apparent, it was indeed significant and interfered with rehabilitation therapies. With a younger post-combat population in the sub-acute phase, psychiatric interviews revealed depression, overwhelming anxieties and emotional instability. However, concurrently, nursing staff described these same patients as having high morale, feeling fine, and experiencing few worries. On Rorschach testing, 50% of these 100 amputees showed signs of serious psychopathology and 81% gave evidence of sexual conflict [16]. In another study [11], amputees who consistently denied any negative affect became agitated when difficulties were brought into consciousness, while the

magical, wishful thinking of others became so exaggerated as to be pathological. When offered an atmosphere of acceptance and support, amputees were
relieved by the opportunity to ventilate and talk about feelings of alienation,
boredom, and powerlessness. Not having to deny distress and appear falsely
cheerful was labeled a great relief. Self-reports of personal grief, fears of losing another limb, anxiety about falling, concern about increased dependency
and discomfort over reactions of non-amputees were common [2, 3, 9, 17,
18].

Chronic Phase

In the chronic phase, also, both traumatic and diseased amputees have
great reluctance to be open and honest about their feelings. *Siller and Silverman* [19], in their post-rehabilitation study of 359 amputees, described a 'collective mask' which their subjects used to present themselves to the public.
On measures relating to acceptance by self and others, sociability, independence, functional adequacy and frustration, amputees consistently describe
themselves as they believed they should be, rather than how they actually
were. Insight into their present situation was gained through study of their
fantasies and wishes, and through observation of the unrealistic expectations
which were maintained. *C.M. Parkes* [13] described the 'stiff upper lip'
adjustment made by his compulsively self-reliant amputees and suggested
that their good outcomes were more apparent than real.

Other studies on long-term adjustment of amputees, while few in numbers, underscore the seriousness of the difficulties, with reports of insecurity,
self-consciousness, restlessness and insomnia. Mean scores on a variety of
indices of depression and anxiety, months and years post-amputation, are
considerably elevated compared to non-amputee populations [2, 13, 20]. A
study of 200 traumatic amputees identified a continuing pattern of resentment or defiance in almost half the subjects [12]. In terms of vocational
behavior, amputees accepting work that was either far too demanding or was
excessively below potential has frequently been noted [12, 13].

Phantom Limb Sensations and Phantom Limb Pain

The psychological sequelae to amputation may be complicated by the
amputee's experience of the phantom limb. Removal of a limb results in the

loss of a complex, coordinated, functional activity which had been integrated into the body scheme [21]. The phantom limb phenomenon is a reflection of an amputee's previous life experiences in sensing, attending and learning in the physical world [22]. Phantom sensations are considered a usual experience post-surgery and a part of the modification of the total body image [23]. In many patients, these sensations disappear with time [24, 25].

Specific psychological dimensions have been linked by some observers to individual experiences of the phantom limb. Levels of conflict and anxiety have been found to be directly related to intensity, persistency and duration of phantom limb sensation [26, 27]. Some researchers [27, 28] have suggested a negative correlation between phantom limb experience and a reorganized self-image, realistic acceptance of the self and satisfactory social adjustment. Others [29, 30], however, have found no relationship among such variables. The persistent phantom sensation has also been conceptionalized as an unresolved grief process in which the body part cannot be experienced as acutally lost. As such, the loss is denied, and the persisting sensations become a wishfulfillment hallucination [31]. Interestingly, amputees may re-experience phantom limb sensations when questioned about emotionally distressing issues or under certain emergency conditions [31, 32].

Some amputees have to contend with both phantom limb sensations and phantom limb pain, the latter an extremely disagreeable sensation often described as twisting, burning, cramping, or pinching. Amputees who report pain have been observed to score higher on neurotic scales [1], show marked psychopathology [27, 33] and have severe personality disturbances [32]. Reported incidence of this phantom limb pain range from 2% to 48% [9, 27, 31, 33]. Both the subjective nature of pain and the lack of careful measurement of its frequency and duration in patients studied may account for conflicting data. *Parkes'* [27] study distinguished between intermittent and continuous phantom pain at four to 8 weeks post-surgery, and again at 13 months. Among 46 amputees, 78% were diseased and 22% injured. Intermittent pain was experienced by 52% initially, with this figure dropping only to 48%; continuous pain began at 7% and decreased to 4% a year later. These results are consistent with *Parkes'* general conclusion that the subacute reactions of the amputee tend to remain relatively unchanged over time.

Controversy persists over the role of both lingering phantom limb sensations and that of phantom limb pain. While biological pain may distort or exaggerate psychological assessment, it has been suggested that phantom pain can be relieved by psychiatric therapies [34]. Persistent phantom sensations and pain are symptoms which suggest closer scrutiny by the examining psychiatrist.

The Role of Life Cycle

Any age-appropriate crisis is a significant factor in an individual's reaction to amputation. For example, a 19 year old accident victim who is already coping with issues related to separation and independence will have special difficulties during the rehabilitation process [35]. While children and adolescents are obvious examples of the interactive effect of developmental issues and other major life events, adults are now also recognized as passing through life stages characterized by intense feelings and requiring adaptive mastery [36]. Recent divorce, death of a loved one or major changes in life work are signal events which alert the clinician to the likelihood of increased coping difficulties. An individual's history of successes and failures may assist the clinician in locating areas of vulnerability which need support and ones of strength which can be maximized.

Grief Work

Grieving is an expected sequelae to the loss of a part of one's body. Somatic components and psychological symptoms include: sighing, tearfulness, anorexia, feelings of weakness, irritability, self-accusation, hostility and preoccupation with the image of the lost object [10, 37]. Grief work involves thinking, feeling and talking about inner responses to the changed body. It results in freedom from attachment to the lost part, readjustment to an environment where the missing part is permanently gone and formation of new outlets to replace functions of the old [11]. Morbid grief represents a transformation of a normal response into delayed or distorted response, such as hyperactivity with no sense of the loss [37]. Impulsive behavior, social withdrawal, the absence of spontaneous attempts at readjustment and lack of cooperation with staff may indicate a blocked grief process [11, 38]. Grieving may extend beyond the actual loss itself to include sadness and anger over specific goals no longer possible. Unexpressed and perhaps unconscious wishes and desires which were linked to the absent body part may be important issues in grief work.

Body Image

The notion of body image is one which has particular relevance in understanding the tasks an amputee faces in coping with the loss of a major body part [39]. Body image is a psychological identity which gradually develops from the interplay of objective and subjective reality throughout the life span of an individual. Sensations and preceptions are the building blocks of body image, but emotional energies direct and interpret this raw material which is organized in highly individualistic ways. Body image issues relate both to a person's pre-surgical sense of self [40] as well as to the specific experiences which result from the surgery. Influences on body image may be experienced as reality, conscious fantasy or unconscious symbolism [23]. Adult body images may retain early symbolic associations from infancy and childhood, with such primitive constructs emerging under the stress of significant body change [14].

Objective reality has changed dramatically for an amputee. During the early days and weeks after surgery, the patient retains a mental picture of the self as a whole, intact person. The individual who absent-mindedly tries to walk on a limb no longer there is experiencing the discrepancy between the former body state and the present actual self. The stimulus pattern of perceptions, sensations and cognition must be re-evaluated and integrated into a new precept [41]. Specific constraints obviously accompany the loss of an arm or a leg. A normal adjustment process consists of a gradual acceptance of the physical realities of the loss with reasonable expectations of future performance. The former body image, i.e., of a person with no missing parts, is modified so that the new image accepts the changed physical state which is now 'normal'.

The subjective meaning of the amputated body part has a direct bearing on the psychological sequelae of the surgery. The value of the lost part depends on the importance of that part to the person's total sense of identity. Typical examples include a lower limb amputee, formerly a construction worker who climbed beams to earn a livelihood, and an artist, whose emotional life was invested in oil painting on canvas before the loss of a hand. Amputations for these individuals created massive disruption in both economic and emotional areas. More subtle examples are a young man whose ability to relate to others was completely dependent on his image as an athlete, and a socially-minded woman whose life was focused on external appearance. These individuals were devastated because loss of body part meant loss of personal worth. The prior life style of these last 2 cases had enabled them to cope successfully with inner insecurities by emphasizing their physical bodies. Change in body appearance destroys this emotional crutch. If there are insufficient inner resources to mobilize other adaptive behaviors, the substitution of new values and goals for old ones may be blocked.

The symbolic meaning of the actual removal of a part of the self is another facet of the body image issue. Fears of annihilation and castration anxieties are commonly linked with amputation. An individual's often unconscious interpretation of the now-altered state may assume forms such as heroic sacrifice, deserved punishment, confirmation of loathsomeness or shameful humiliation [14, 23]. Thorough history taking and attention to the patient's free associations regarding the amputation may uncover the roots of exaggerated or distorted thinking.

The internal struggles of a new amputee are compounded by the reactions of family, friends and the public who may experience confusion, discomfort, and uncertainty about how to behave toward the person with a missing body part [42]. Other negative feelings experienced by both family and the public are active aversion and disgust. Non-amputee onlookers may be fascinated by, and yet afraid of, a person with a missing limb. Such powerful feelings presumably reflect unconscious fears of incorporation of the mutilated body image into the observer's own self. The physical and/or emotional withdrawal of others jeopardizes the amputee's ongoing personal and professional relationships, while the stigma itself may result in reduced social status. Such conditions make the amputee ripe for personal and vocational exploitation. The most damaging outcome for the amputee is the possible incorporation of the negative responses of others into the individual's own esteem system [1, 6, 11].

Prosthesis

The adjustment work an amputee faces may be ameliorated by successful use of a prosthesis. Almost all recent amputees, regardless of age or state of health, want an artificial limb [43, 44]. A prosthesis can provide visual and/or functional replacement for the amputated limb. An objective sense of disability is often related to participation in activities, and for the lower limb amputee, there is a dramatic distinction between those who can walk and those who cannot [1].

A prosthesis would seem to help restore completeness of body image on emotional as well as physical levels. For some patients, it may even be treasured as a substitute for the loss of a precious belonging [12]. The value of the prosthesis to the amputee depends on the degree to which it is integrated into the body scheme [28]. Reports of feeling naked without one's artificial limb verify a successfully integrated prosthetic device [1].

The enthusiasm of staff and recent amputees for prostheses contrasts with data on the long-term use of the device. *Mazet's* study [44] of 1770 lower limb amputees over a ten-year period found that more than $\frac{1}{2}$ discarded the artificial limb within 6 months. An English study identified this same 50% rate of use of lower limb prostheses on 341 subjects [45]. When above-the-knee were separated from below-the-knee amputees, the use rate for above-the-knee amputees dropped to 15–25% [3, 4, 46]. Continued use of upper extremity prostheses have not been carefully evaluated.

A number of factors influence whether or not a prosthesis is used successfully for an extended period. The *Kay and Pennal* study [43] matched subjects on age and proficiency of use and concluded that psychological factors were responsible for early discard of the device. *Mazet* [44] related failure in his study to body image conflicts and the inability of some amputees to alter their self-perception in order to include the prosthetic device. The 50% rate of use in the *McKenzie* study [45] was unusually high, considering the amputees were all over 65. Success was attributed to the particular prosthetic center which stressed global patient assessment with consideration of the patient's physical, mental and emotional make-up, as well as the nature of the environment to which the amputee would return.

Long-term succesful use of a prosthesis is dependent on a number of variables which relate to psychological as well as physical factors. The discarding of a prosthesis does not necessarily indicate psychological maladjustment. The specific reality of each amputee is an important consideration.

Intervention Strategies

Because of the multiplicity of problems presented by amputation, virtually all recent amputees can profit from some type of psychological support. The most frequently mentioned therapeutic intervention is that of peer group meetings, most of which are structured primarily for education, social support, role modeling and sharing of experiences [2, 3, 47]. Another type of

intervention is group therapy for amputees. While many supporters pro-
claimed these groups as highly successful, others found such therapy not
appropriate because of dependent and regressive attitudes fostered by the
traumatic experience of amputation [26]. (Outcome evaluations of psychological interventions in surgical patients is discussed on p. 23.)

Short-term individual psychotherapy is recommended by some practi-
tioners [9, 13, 16]. *Kolb* [34] believed that intensive treatment was necessary
in order to modify pathological and unconscious meanings of body structure
change. He suggested a brief therapeutic intervention with focus on: phantom limb sensation and any rationalizations about it; wishes and fears about
disposal of the body part; and past and present attitudes toward the body in
relation to real or fantasized experiences with significant others. Clinical lore
indicates that psychotherapeutic work must include appropriate gentle confrontation and solid support of the patient's defensive structure. Sexual
counseling may be limited to practical concerns or may extend to latent fears
about potency and desirability.

Assisting the amputee in dealing with interactional tensions with non-
amputees may be appropriate [48]. Interviews with significant others may
provide important information as to environmental stresses the amputee is
experiencing. Feelings of family members which relate to dependency needs,
sexual concerns and any suggestion of active aversion or morbid preoccupation with the surgery should be carefully assessed. Therapeutic value may
result from helping significant others to identify and label their thoughts
and feelings. Follow-up work with the amputee may be partially guided by
knowledge of the very real tensions which will be confronted on a daily
basis.

Conclusion

Many amputees eventually overcome the multiple hurdles which are
posed by the loss of a major body part, while others are not so successful. A
noted clinician, *L. Friedmann,* has stated quite frankly, 'treating the psychological problems faced by the amputee often has more significance to his life
than the quality of the surgery or the nature of prosthetic device' [1]. Psychosocial intervention early in the rehabilitation process can be seen as a form
of primary prevention, with ultimate benefits to patient, family and the
society to which the amputee returns.

References

1   Friedmann, L.: The psychological rehabilitation of the amputee (Charles C. Thomas, Springfield, Ill., 1978).

2   MacBride, A.; Rogers, J.; Whylie, B.; Freeman, S.: Psychosocial factors in the rehabilitation of elderly amputees. Psychosom. *21*(3): 258–265 (1980).

3   Rogers, J.; MacBride, A.; Whylie, B.; Freeman, S.: The use of groups in the rehabilitation of amputees. Int. J. Psychiat. *8*(3): 243–255 (1977–78).

4   Brown, P.: Rehabilitation of bilateral lower extremity amputees. J. Bone Joint Surg. *52A*(4): 687–700 (1970).

5   National Research Council. The Geriatric amputee: Principles of management. National Academy of Sciences, Washington, D.C., 1971.

6   Fishman, S.: Amputation; in: Garrett, J., Levine, F. (eds), Psychological practices with the physically disabled, pp. 1–50 (Columbia University Pess, New York, 1962).

7   Kelham, R.: Some thoughts on the mental effects of amputation. Brit. Med. J. *1*: 334–337 (1958).

8   Arnold, H.: Elderly diabetic amputees. Am. J. Nursing *67*: 2646 (1969).

9   Caplan, L.; Hackett, T.: Emotional effects of lower limb amputation in the aged. New Engl. J. Med. *269*: 1166–1191 (1963).

10 Parkes, C.: Components of the reaction to loss of a limb, spouse or home. J. Psychosom. Res. *16*: 343–349 (1972).

11 Frank, J.: Amputee war casualty in a military hospital: observations on psychological management. Int. J. Psychiat. Med. *4*(1): 1–16 (1973).

12 Wittkower, E.: Rehabilitation of the limbless: joint surgical and psychological study. Occupat. Med. *3*: 20–44 (1947).

13 Parkes, C.: The psychological reaction to loss of a limb: the first year after amputation; in Howells, Modern perspectives in the psychiatric aspects of surgery, pp. 515–532 (Brunner/Mazel, New York, 1976).

14 Braceland, F.: Role of the psychiatrist in rehabilitation. J. Am. Med. Ass. *165*: 211–215 (1957).

15 Goin, J.; Goin, M.K.: Changing the body: psychological effects of plastic surgery. (Williams & Wilkins, Baltimore, Md. 1981).

16 Randall, G.; Ewalt, J.; Blair, H.: Psychiatric reactions to amputation. J. Am. Med. Ass. *128*(9): 645–652 (1945).

17 Fisher, W.; Samuelson, C.: Group psychotherapy for selected patients with lower extremity amputations. Arch. Phys. Med. Rehabil. *52*(1): 79 (1971).

18 Freeman, A.; Applegate, W.: Psychiatric consultation to a rehabilitation program for amputees. Hosp. Comm. Psychiat. *27*: 40–42 (1976).

19 Siller, J.; Silverman, S.: Studies of upper extremity amputees: psychological factors. Artif. Limbs *5*(2): 88–116 (1958).

20 Lundberg, S.G.: Body image disturbance and lower limb amputation: Masters thesis, UTHSCD 1983.

21 Rubin, R.: Body image and self-esteem. Nursing Outl. *6*: 20–22 (1968).

22 Fisher, R.: Out on a (phantom) limb. Persp. Biol. Med. *12*(2): 259–272 (1964).

23 Kolb, L.: Disturbances of the body image; in Arieti, I. ed., American handbook of psychiatry, No. 1, (Basic Books Inc., New York 1959).

24 Carlen, P.; Wall, P.; Nadvorna, H.; Steinbach, T.: Phantom limb and related phenomena

in recent traumatic amputation. Neurology *28*(3): 211–217 (1978).

25   Soloman, G.; Schmidt, K.: A burning issue: phantom limb pain and psychological preparation of the patient for amputation. Arch. Surg. *13:* 185–186 (1978).

26   Noble, D.; Price, D.; Gilder, R.: Psychiatric disturbances following amputation. Am. J. Psychiat. *110*(2): 609–613 (1954).

27   Parkes, C.: Factors determining the persistence of phantom pain in the amputee. J. Psychosom. Res. *17:* 97–108 (1973).

28   Weiss, S.: The body image as related to phantom sensation: a hypothetical conceptualization of seemingly isolated findings. Ann. New York Acad. Science *74:* 25–29 (1958).

29   Almagor, M.; Jaffe, Y.; Lomranz, J.: The relation between limb dominance, acceptance of disability and the phantom limb phenomenon. J. Abnorm. Psychol. *87*(8): 377–379 (1978).

30   Hirschenfang, F.; Benton, J.: Assessment of phantom limb sensation among patients with lower extremity amputations. J. Psychiat. *63*(2): 197–199 (1966).

31   Kolb, L.: Psychology of the amputee: phantom phenomena, body image and pain. Coll. pap. Mayo Clin. *44:* 586 (1952).

32   Simmel, M.: On phantom limbs. Arch. Neurol. Psychiat. *75:* 637–647 (1956).

33   Ewalt, J.; Randall, G.; Morris, H.: Phantom limb: Interpretation and significance. Psychosom. Med. *9:* 118–123 (1947).

34   Kolb, L.: Psychiatric aspects of treatment for intractable pain in the phantom limb. Med. Clin. North Am. *4:* 1029–1041 (1950).

35   Wilson, P.: Coping with amputation; 135th APA Annual Meeting, (Toronto, Canada 1982).

36   Sheey, G.: Passages: Predictable crisis of adult life. (E.P. Dutton, New York 1976).

37   Lindemann, E.: Asymptomatology and management of acute grief. Am. J. Psych. *101:* 141–148 (1944).

38   Rosen, V.: The role of denial in acute postoperative affective reactions following removal of body parts. Psychosom. Med. *12.* 356–361 (1950).

39   Lundberg, S.G.; Guggenheim, F.G.: Body image representation in lower limb amputees. (Manuscript in preparation.)

40   Schilder, P.: The image and appearance of the human body. (International Universities Press, New York 1950.)

41   McDaniel, J.: Physical disability and human behavior. (Pergamon Press, New York 1969.)

42   Dembo, T.; Leviton, G.; Wright, B.: Adjustment to misfortune. Art. Limbs *3*(1): 12–65 (1956).

43   Kay, G.; Pennal, G.: Rehabilitation of the elderly amputee. Can. J. Surg. *2:* 44–51 (1958).

44   Mazet, R.: The geriatric amputee. Art. Limbs *11*(2): 33–41 (1967).

45   McKenzie, D.: The elderly amputee. Brit. Med. J. *1:* 153–156 (1953).

46   Burgess, E.; Romano, R.; Zettl, J.; Schrock, R.: Amputations of the leg for peripheral vascular insufficiency. J. Bone Joint Surg. *53A*(5): 874–889 (1971).

47   Lipp, M.; Malone, S.: Rehabilitation of vascular surgery patients. Arch. Phys. Med. Rehabil. *57:* 180–183 (1976).

48   Chaikin, H.; Warfield, M.: Stigma management and amputee rehabilitation. Rehabil. Lit. *34*(6): 162–166 (1973).

Sherry G. Lundberg, MS, Instructor, Richland College, Dallas, TX 75200 (USA)

Adv. psychosom. Med., vol. 15, pp. 211–225 (Karger, Basel 1986)

Penile Prostheses: A Psychiatric Perspective

Thomas D. Stewart

Assistant Professor of Psychiatry Harvard Medical School and Director, Consultation/Liaison Service, Beth Israel Hospital, Boston, Mass., USA

Thus the body speaks [1].

A man is impotent. He receives a message from his body, as does his partner. Is this malfunction a metaphor expressing a more pervasive limpness of character? Is the gauge for measuring physical and emotional health saying something? His partner may speculate: does he want me; is he angry with me? Doubt, anxiety, and frustration – a cornucopia of concerns – permeate the man and his intimate relationships. Wouldn't an unfailing phallus be a perfect solution to this problem? That question is the topic of this paper.

The definition of impotence is arbitrary. Primary impotence has been defined by *Masters and Johnson* as the inability to maintain an erection sufficient for coital connection at any point in a man's life, whereas secondary impotence is present when there is a failure rate of 25% following successful coital approaches [2]. The prevalence for these two conditions is estimated at 1% but may be much higher [3]. Many men suffer in silence.

Freud made one of the first careful explorations of the psychodynamic underpinnings of erectile dysfunction [4]. He focused on the confusion which may exist in a man's mind between his mother and his lover. By becoming impotent he avoids an unconsciously forbidden act. Psychotherapy unfortunately has not been too successful in helping men unravel this dilemma so that they can enjoy their available partner in the present. Failure rates as high as 60% have been cited [5]. Behaviorally oriented approaches emphasizing desensitization in conjunction with sensate focus have reduced the failure rate to a more respectable 41% for primary impotence and 31% for secondary impotence [2]. Psychogenic impotence and organic impotence are both conditions to be considered for penile implant.

Before operating on a man's penis, urologists undertake a thorough clinical assessment of their patient and hopefully the significant other [6, 7]. This study usually includes careful psychiatric and psychological examination [8, 9]. Many facets of human behavior, function, and malfunction are considered. Basic components of the physiological work-up will be reviewed. This chapter will conclude with considerations of treatment options, post-operative outcome studies and a comparison of the pros and cons of each prosthetic device.

Surgical Procedures

In the early part of this century, diverse surgical procedures were used to relieve impotence [10]. In the 1920's bilateral vasectomy and testicular transplantation were heralded as successful, possibly due to transient increases in testosterone levels. Ligation of the dorsal vein of the penis was done to reduce venous outflow. All these efforts, however, failed the test of time. The first surgical implants were done in the 1930's, with rib cartilage used for rigidity. Unfortunately, the results were transient, for the rib cartilage warps in 18 months and then dissolves. Bony erectile augmentation is not unusual in animals. Dogs, bears, and wolves all possess an os penis. The oosik, a walrus penile bone, is of such dimension and mass that it can be confused with a human femur. Some whales have similar erectile assists, raising a question of how unnatural prostheses actually are, considering this occurrence in the animal world.

Contemporary technical developments involving inert synthetic materials, along with advances in surgical techniques over the past 15 years, have made penile prostheses an increasingly useful option in the treatment of impotence. There are 2 types: the inflatable prosthesis and the silastic semi-erect.

The *Scott* prosthesis is the most widely used inflatable model. Introduced in the late 1960's, subsequent modifications have been made to improve reliability [3, 11–13]. Installation of this prosthesis involves the placement of a radio opaque liquid-filled reservoir in the abdomen outside the peritoneal space but under the abdominal musculature. This reservoir connects to a pump in the scrotum which can move the fluid from the reservoir to 2 inflatable cylinders placed in the corpora cavernosa. After use the patient releases the valve in the pump, allowing the fluid to return to the reservoir.

Semi-rigid implants occur in several forms. 3 of the more common are the Small-Carrion, the Jonas, and the Finney. The Small involves placement of two semi-rigid silastic rods into the corpora cavernosa, thus maintaining the penis in a semi-erect state [14]. The Jonas is a modification involving the placement of flexible strands of silver twisted wire in the center of the silastic rods so it can be moved into position for use as needed [15]. The Finney is hinged so it can be locked into position for insertion [16].

Medical Disorders Associated with Impotence

These devices have been used to treat patients suffering from a wide range of conditions which are united only in their ability to cause impotence. These conditions include diabetes mellitus, multiple sclerosis, spinal cord injury, Peyronies Disease and penile amputation [17–23]. Other medical causes of impotence include sleep apnea, prostatitis, urethritis and phimosis. Surgical procedures followed by impotence include: second renal transplants, (probably secondary to disruption of pelvic arterial supply [24]), prostatectomy, sphincterectomy, bowel resection and trauma surgery [24, 26, 27]. Caution has been urged regarding some surgical intervention since spontaneous recovery of erections occurs up to twelve months post retransplant [29]. Prostheses have also found increased use in psychogenic impotence when the problem persists despite extended psychotherapeutic endeavors [28].

Should climax and/or ejaculation have been possible before implantation, as is often the case with diabetes, these functions will continue and possibly be enhanced post-operatively. In some conditions benefits go beyond increased sexual functioning. For example, a prosthesis will allow a normal urine stream post penile amputation, and in spinal cord injury the prosthesis will allow easier use of condom drainage [30]. A normal urine stream and fewer condom accidents provide psychological benefits that speak for themselves.

Neurophysiology of Erection

Understanding the assessment of erectile function requires a brief review of the neurophysiology of erection [31, 32]. Erection reflects an interplay of endocrine, vascular, and neurologic functions. Disruption at any point in these 3 areas can cause impotence. Endocrine function is vital for erections since low testosterone or high prolactin levels will produce impotence. Many questions remain concerning the neurophysiology of erections, including the putative existence of polsters.

Neurologic Component

The neurologic component can be divided into several sections. Cognition, perception and fantasy interconnect in the limbic system with affects and memories to provide input to the penis, mediated by the thoraco-lumbar sympathetic outflow in conjunction with parasympathetic connections from S 2, 3 and 4. The tragedy of spinal cord injuries has helped to clarify the neural mechanisms of erection. Spastic patients with complete cord injury often have reflex erections resulting from upper motor neuron disinhibition. Flaccid cord-injured patients with complete levels below (T-12) have no reflex erections but may have psychogenic erections derived from thought and fantasy, thus connecting the thoraco-lumbar innervation with the cortical component of erections.

To determine if a neurologic component exists in a patient with possible neurogenic impotency, cystometry sometimes is used.

Vascular Component

Erection, a vascular phenomenon, occurs when arterioles flow into latent vascular sponge-like spaces in the corpora cavernosa. 'Polsters' are thought to exist which function as valves under autonomic control from the thoracolumbar and sacral areas. In the flaccid state the polsters shunt arterial blood into penile veins. Under erotic stimulation the polsters close, blocking direct access to the penile veins, thus forcing blood flow into the cavernous spaces. The blood supply for erections comes from the internal pudendal arteries which are branched from the internal iliac arteries. A non-invasive technique to investigate vascular disease is the Doppler probe. Penile arterial flow and penile blood pressure can be detected with the aid of a pediatric blood pressure cuff. Vascular occlusive disease can sometimes be pinpointed with this device. Cavernosography to determine adequacy to cavernous filling may sometimes be required [34].

Endocrinologic Components

Endocrine dysfunction anywhere along the hypothalamic-pituitary-gonadal axis may present as impotence [33]. *Spark*, an endocrinologist, studied 105 consecutive patients referred to him for impotence. 37 (35%) had abnormalities of the hypothalamic-pituitary-gonadal axis. 20 had hypogonadotropic hypogonadism with Luteinizing Hormone (LH) levels below normal. 7 suffered from hypergonadotrophic hypogonadism reflecting end organ unresponsiveness to adequate LH levels. Hyperprolactinemia was evident in 8 and hyperthyroidism in 2 cases.

One screening test result, a low serum testosterone, would have detected endocrine dysfunction in 36 of these 37 men. One of these men had a normal testosterone with hyperprolactinemia. Correction of the endocrine imbalance restored erectile function in 31 of the 37. While this study does not purport to be a random survey, it does support the consideration of endocrine malfunction in the assessment of impotence with at least the determination of a serum testosterone.

Other Assessment of Organic Component

Several recent technical developments have helped to pinpoint organic contributions to impotence, which may be multiple. The most well known of these in nocturnal penile tumescence (NPT) monitoring, introduced by *Karacan* [36, 37]. Strain gauges are attached to the penis with transducers that allow recordings of penile expansion during sleep. The assumption is that men with psychogenic impotence will show normal erections during sleep, whereas those with organic dysfunction will continue to not have erections while sleeping.

Pharmacological Agents Associated with Impotence

Medications can cause a variety of sexual dysfunctions, including impotence. Anticholinergic drugs, such as some antidepressants and antipsychotics, are common causes of impotence, as are some antihypertensives. Sometimes a simple change in medication can provide relief. *Lipson* studied 264 hypertensive diabetic men who were taking hydrochlorothiazide along with either clonidine or alpha methyl dopa as their secondary anti-hypertensive drug. 60% were impotent [35]. By changing to prazosin as the secondary drug, 79% reported 'substantial improvement' in sexual function. While neither blind nor controlled, the study underlines the importance of medication review, even in a population whose impotence could easily be explained by diabetes.

Alcohol in excess is probably the most common pharmacological agent to cause impotence. Acute sexual dysfunction after drinking is an occasional occurrence for many men. Peripheral neuropathy following chronic alcohol abuse can make this problem permanent.

The importance of medical knowledge to assist in determining the suitability of a man for a prosthesis is evident. This decision involves a confluence of physiologic and psychologic functional considerations where the psychiatrist's medical background is especially relevant. An interview utilizing the full array of a psychiatrist's psychotherapeutic and medical skills is a key diagnostic tool which will now be considered.

Psychological Considerations

Impotence is a deflating experience in every sense of the word. Psychiatric evaluation before prosthesis implantation provides an opportunity to explore the experience and its meaning. Such an interview not only gathers information but also allows the patient to have a potential healing experience as he shares his hurt for what may be the first time [8]. This initial discussion of the interview assumes that the patient has been determined by previously described tests as organically impotent or has suffered from psychogenic impotence refractory to psychotherapeutic intervention.

Appreciation of the phenomenology of the patient's impotence can help him and the psychiatrist gain perspective regarding his desires to undergo this sometimes painful and frightening procedure which involves cutting into his genitals. Memories like envying another man as he buys a large supply of condoms or bumbling explanations to a disappointed partner can be elicited. In short, ask, 'What has this been like for you?'

The fact of impotence can generalize into a more pervasive sense of ineffectiveness [38]. A weak penis can become for the patient a visible symbol for the invisible feeling of global impotence and can evolve into a metaphor. Sadistic humor, along with the commonplace usage of the word 'impotence' describing such diverse issues as foreign policy and personality style, can reinforce this metaphor. The extent of this generalization must be addressed by doctor and patient, since this inner sense can persist after the deficit itself is operatively corrected. Post-operative psychotherapy may be indicated to help a man discover that penile dysfunction need not preclude potent behavior.

Depression can be viewed as a reflection of the gap between expectations and reality. Pointed questioning about benefits anticipated from prosthesis placement are in order. If fantasies about post-operative life can be discovered and reality tested by the urologist or psychiatrist, some discouragement can be avoided. An example would be the man who expected his feelings to change because his penis did. His self-esteem may improve, but it might not.

There are other hidden hopes that may be present. Some potential recipients reason, 'it will make her respond'. A man said this to the author, although further questioning revealed the couple was not even holding hands and barely talked. Couples work was suggested. Some spinal cord patients in the author's experience had the magical thought that operatively-restored erections would mean return of fertility and orgastic experience. Clarifying this was always sad for both parties.

Ferreting out hidden agendas helps, but unrealistic hopes may remain. Underselling the benefits of penile implants can reduce the stimulation of hopes that may never be realized or even expressed.

Some pre-operative referrals may be for a determination of whether or not impotence is psychogenic. Such an assessment should emphasize the detection of anxiety, especially in sexual settings, and the presence of depression or psychosis. Traditional psychiatric questioning should suffice with modifications to emphasize the connection between dysphoric states and sexual activity.

Gauging of depression and anxiety is rendered difficult by the very presence of impotence – which is not known for its favorable effect on self-esteem. For example, loss of libido is a vegetative sign. Recurrent impotence, though, can undermine the urge to connect sexually. Repeated failure is the ideal inhibitor of the wish to try anything sexual or not. Sex-related anxiety is equally difficult to assess. Who wouldn't become anxious, anticipating failure? The only way out of the above bind is to clarify carefully the man's emotional state when impotence first became a problem, assuming it has not been lifelong. However, onset is often gradual with intermittent potency, both complete and partial, blurring the delineation of an emotional baseline.

Psychogenic or Organic Impotence, Based on Interview

There are specific questions that help sort out psychogenic and organic contributions, but some of these are a good deal more helpful than others. The most obvious is asking whether or not there are conditions (e.g. masturbation) where potency and ejaculation are consistently present.

Abel has developed a set of 7 sexual symptoms (SSS) which can be obtained from an interview [39]. These serve as a screening device to determine if NPT monitoring would be useful. 100% rigid erection is used to define potency in an effort to avoid ambiguity about the meaning of potency. A positive answer to all 7 was 100% sensitive in finding organic impotence (all organic impotence found) and 76% chance that a man found organically impotent by these questions would have it confirmed by NPT monitoring.

These 7 symptoms are delineated by responses to the following statements:

---

1. Everytime I try to get an erection it is less than a 100% full erection.
2. I never wake up in the morning or during the night with a 100% full erection.
3. It frequently or always takes me longer to reach ejaculation than it used to.
4. During oral sex or masturbation I always get less than 100% full erection.
5. The amount I ejaculate is frequently or always less than it used to be.
6. I rarely or never ejaculate prematurely (too soon).
7. I frequently or always fail to get a 100% full erection.

These 7 were selected from a list of relevant questions. Several other items that were not helpful in differential diagnosis were: the presence of partial erections 100% of the time, the absence of stress at the onset of impotence, and lack of partner specificity for the impotence.

There are several caveats regarding *Abel's* work which he points out. The patients were all diabetic. Similar results might not be obtained if other problems were included. 41% of the patient (N = 60) in this study fell into a 'cannot call' category. Equally discouraging was *Abel's* follow up of clinical interviews by NPT monitoring. 50% of the clinical diagnoses (organic, psychogenic, or cannot call) had to be changed following the sleep laboratory studies regardless of the SSS and NPT findings; many still could not be diagnosed definitively. Finally, this format has not been replicated.

The Minnesota Multiphasic Personality Inventory, the Male Impotence Test and the Derogatis Sexual Functioning Inventory all looked quite promising for the delineation of organicity and psychogenicity but did not stand up well replication was attempted [39].

In the author's view, an interview with the significant other, if there is one, is a vital part of the complete assessment. *Gee*, however, feels that such contact should be made only if the urologist deems this necessary [40]. Untoward experiences have occurred even when a spouse has been carefully evaluated. For example, one such woman left her husband promptly after he came home with his new inflatable prosthesis [41]. At the other extreme, women have been reported who were pleased with their man's new found potency, being unaware a device had been installed [42].

Should psychogenic dysfunction be a question, discussion with spouse could help determine the role of couple's problems in the difficulty. Even if the impotence is organic beyond a doubt, the value of asking the recipient for her views and concerns about receiving this device speaks for itself since the loss and suffering associated with impotence is shared. The fear of injury deserves attention as do her expectations of what a prosthesis will do for them. In one study less than one half of female partners were even advised that sexual activity with a prosthesis in place would not harm her vagina or damage his penis [43]. Of interest is the manner in which Scott's team at Baylor evaluates the sexual partner. The assessing psychiatrist uses a questionnaire with the patient which 'gathers information about the patient's personality, his sexual relations, and the personality of his spouse or sexual partner' [9]. This represents a novel approach to understanding a person without the aid of an interview. Wouldn't she be the best source of information about herself?

Suitability for Penile Prosthesis

Recent developments complicate the decision to place a prosthesis and cast into a different perspective some of the data previously presented. Penile prostheses are now used in men with known psychogenic impotence which has been intractable to psychotherapeutic interventions and the passage of time. Thus the diagnosis of psychogenic dysfunction in itself is not a contraindication to the use of a prosthesis.

Furthermore, the established presence of organic impotence does not rule out effective behavioral intervention in the resumption of functional erections. As part of extensive investigations into endocrine function, NPT and diabetes, *Ficher* et al. uncovered some interesting findings [44]. They gave 50 couples sensate focus therapy similar to that of *Masters and Johnson* [45]. All males had diabetes and had impotence established secondary to related pathophysiology. In 23 cases, successful vaginal penetration was achieved and in the 27 unsuccessful (by that measure) efforts, the man's feelings about sex often improved. *Bohannon* also used brief sensate focus therapy, averaging 7 sessions to help 28 of 34 diabetic men self-referred for impotence to achieve vaginal intromission [46]. This study lacked NPT monitoring to help determine physiologic competence. Thus these encouraging results could reflect success with men whose problems were primarily emotional.

Choice of Surgical Implants

Once the decision to install a prosthesis has been made, the urologist and patient review the pros and cons of each device as well as potential complications [47]. While detailed knowledge of these issues is beyond the purview of a psychiatrist's role, some familiarity with these facts is in order. The Small-Carrion (silastic implant), Finney (hinged silastic) and the Jonas (silastic with a braided wire core) offer several advantages over the inflatable prostheses.

The silastic models are simpler and quicker to install than the Scott (inflatable). Operative time can be as low as 45 minutes versus 2 hours for the Scott Cost, which includes the device and the hospital stay, is less as well: $2,000–3,000 for the silastic implants versus $5,000–8,000 for the Scott [48, 49]. Urologists in India have reduced costs to a bare minimum by placing a silastic rod into only one of the two corpora cavernosa with apparently good results [50]. Should the prosthesis be undesirable for any reason, silastic implants are much easier to remove with the extraction often being done on an outpatient basis.

The Scott may require up to a week admission as opposed to 2–3 days for silastic models, with some silastic implants done on an outpatient basis. Some centers, however, have drastically reduced the hospital stay and operative time for inserting the Scott.

Simplicity and economy, however, are not the only considerations. A man with the Scott has a more natural appearance while erect. Placement of his penis is no problem once deflated, whereas his counterpart with a semi-rigid device may need to avoid tight pants and fold his penis against his abdomen to keep his erection from showing. The silastic continuous semi-erect state carries a greater risk of urethral erosion and may render subsequent cystoscopy more difficult. The Scott, of course, avoids these pitfalls, but unfortunately often requires revision due to mechanical failure. The current rate of reoperation is about 20% [3]. Improvements in the valves and hydraulic system are steadily increasing the reliability.

Outcome Studies

All implants usually allow resumption of sexual activity in 4 weeks. Findings in outcome studies vary according to whether men or their partners are queried. Problems with the definition of a favorable outcome abound and most replies must simply be taken at face value. Seeking information about women's reactions to the Small-Carrion prosthesis, Kramarsky-Binkhorst contacted 60 implant recipients: 31 allowed their partner to be interviewed, the others refusing because of non-use or fears about the stability of their relationship [43]. Less than one half of the partners were satisfied with the results. The most serious complaints involved concerns about size and rigidity. 'It was believed to be to short, to thick, to flexible and that it buckled at the top making vaginal penetration or effective containment impossible.'

As part of a study at the Joslin Clinic, 107 impotent diabetic men had prostheses installed, 85% of which were the Small-Carrion design [17]. 91 (84%) agreed to participate in the questionnaire study. 81% of those responding would again choose to have the implant; 12% were equivocal; and 7% would not, citing pain, bulk, and unnaturalness. 70% reported an increase in physical enjoyment along with no overall change in the importance of sex in their lives. 60% of the men who agreed to participate allowed their partners to respond to the questionnaire. 83% of the partners were satisfied, which finding was highly congruent with patient responses. Of interest, only 2 out of 3 sexual partners were asked about the implant pre-operatively. Of those men who did ask their partners, just 66% of the patients said they considered their partner's reply in making their decision.

Other studies have been encouraging. *Scott* indicated that 234 of 235 of his patients were able to use inflatable prosthesis 'to their satisfaction' [3]. *Seagraves* carefully studied 15 patients, 8 of whom received a Scott and the rest, a Small-Carrion [51]. 13 of the 15 had organic impotence. All were pleased and indicated they would undergo the same procedure again. *Seagraves* noted that, '...most men had a degree of restoration of self esteem after surgery...' though the incidence of this change and the means of assessing it were not specified. Unlike most studies, an effort was made to measure coital frequencies which were described as 'reasonable', averaging once per week. *Seagraves* also wrote, 'adverse consequences to the recipients of prostheses were noteworthy by their absence'. His encouraging findings may be colored by the stringent screening program which approved fewer than one in 10 for implant surgery.

Smith compared the outcome of Scott versus Small-Carrion implants [52]. 28 patients were involved, of whom 17 had a Scott. 26 of 28, 'felt more virile and have had greater self-esteem since the operation'. The means of measuring self-esteem was not explained. Over half of the patients in each group had partial erections pre-operatively which continued post-operatively to further enhance their potency. While prosthesis brochures warn that implant placement may destroy pre-existing erectile function, no mention was made of whether this untoward event occurred. Indeed, in no study reviewed for this chapter was decreased erectile capacity secondary to surgery discussed. Cosmetic results, sexual performance and embarrassment about having such a device did not vary significantly for the 2 groups. *Smith* concluded that the patient's attitude had more to do with outcome than device selection.

Surprising results have been noted as well. One man refused to inflate his device due to psychic conflict unresponsive to psychotherapy. Another rarely inflated his because his natural erections improved considerably post-operatively. He explained, 'just knowing it's there is enough for me to function' [53].

The percentage of men who virtually never use their penile prosthesis may be significant, but is not known with certainty. The *Joslin* study found only 2% were non-users, but others have suggested the figure is much higher [17, 42]. Some men will elect neither operative nor psychotherapeutic intervention.

Conclusions

The consulting psychiatrist can make a number of suggestions to impotent patients considering an implant. First, the patient can be supported in efforts to offset the tendency to generalize his deficit. Having erections and being a potent person are not one and the same thing. Second, discussion can be encouraged with the sexual partner to help reduce her feeling that she caused the problem, compounding an already difficult situation. If orgasms are possible in the impotent male, partners should both share in this knowledge since they both may have equated potency and orgastic function. The psychiatrist can directly question the partners about sexual preferences, to increase the likelihood of a rewarding experiences for both without erections. In essence, there are many ways to make love.

From the foregoing information it is clear that penile prostheses can offer an increasingly viable alternative for impotent men. Both operative techniques and technical refinements have steadily evolved over the last 15 years. These improvements have reduced operative time and post-operative morbidity while increasing the likelihood of a favorable outcome. Yet these are not for every man. Some men prefer to love with what they naturally have.

References

1   Mushatt, C.: Mind body environment: Toward understanding the impact of loss on psyche and soma. Psychoanal. Quart. *44:* 81–106 (1975).

2   Masters, W.; Johnson, V.: Human Sexual Inadequacy (Little Brown and Company, Boston 1970).

3   Scott, F.; Byrd, G.; Karacan, I.; Olsson, P.; Beutler, L.; Atlia, S.: Erectile impotence treated with an implantable, inflatable prosthesis. J. Am. Med. Ass. *241:* 2609–2612 (1979).

4   Freud, S.: Contributions to the psychology of love. The most prevalent form of degradation in erotic life. (1912). Collected Papers of Sigmund Freud. Vol. IV, pp. 203–217, (Hogarth Press, London 1949).

5   Cooper, A.: A factual study of male potency disorders. Brit. J. Psychiat. *114:* 719–730 (1968).

6   Montague, D.: Clinical evaluation of impotence. Urol. Clin. North Am. *8:* 103–118 (1981).

7   Morgan, J.; Pryon, J.: The investigation of organic impotence. Brit. J. Urol. *52:* 571–574 (1980).

8   Osborne, D.: Psychological aspects of male sexual dysfunction. Urol. Clin. North Am. *8:* 135–142 (1980).

9   Beutler, L.; Scott, F.; Karacan, I.: Psychological screening of impotent men. J. Urol. *116:* 193–197 (1976).

10   Gee, W.: A history of surgical treatment of impotence. Urology *5:* 40–1405 (1975).

11   Furlow, W.: Surgical management of impotence using the inflatable penile prosthesis. Brit. J. Urol. *50:* 114–117 (1978).

12   Malloy, T.; Wein, A.; Carpiniello, A.: Further experience with the inflatable penile prosthesis. J. Urol. *122:* 478–480 (1979).

13   Scott, F.; Bradley, W.; Timm, B.: Management of erectile impotence. Use of the implantable, inflatable prosthesis. Urology *2:* 80 (1973).

14   Small, M.; Carrion, H.; Gordon, J.: Small-Carrion penile prosthesis. Urology *5:* 479 (1975).

15   Krane, R.; Friedberg, P.; Siroky, M.: Jones silicone silver penile prosthesis: initial experience in America. J. Urol. *126:* 475–476 (1981).

16   Finney, R.: New hinged silicone penile implant. J. Urol. *118:* 585 (1977).

17   Beaser, R.; Van der Hoek, C.; Jacobson, A.; Flood, T.; Desautals, R.: Experience with penile prostheses in the diabetic man. J. Am. Med. Ass. *248:* 943–948 (1982).

18   Burkholder, G.; Nuvell, M.: Amelioration of problems of partial penile amputation. J. Urol. 122: 562–563 (1979).

19   Golgi, H.: Experience with penile prosthesis in spinal cord injury patients. J. Urol. *121:* 288–289 (1979).

20   Krosnick, A.; Podolsky, S.: Diabetes and sexual dysfunction: restoring normal ability. Geriatrics *36:* 92–93 (1981).

21   Massey, E.; Plut, A.: Penile prosthesis for impotence in multiple sclerosis. Ann. Neurol. *6:* 450–452 (1979).

22   O'Donnel, P.: Marlex replacement of unica albuginea. J. Urol. *124:* 732–733 (1980).

23   Alomar, T.; Halikiopoulus, H.; Ragu, T.: Evolution of the surgical management of Peyronies disease. J. Urol. *123:* 680–682 (1980).

24   Burns, J.; Houttuin, E.; Gregory, J.; Hamatmoh, I.; Sullivan, T.: Vascular induced erectile impotence in renal transplant.

25   Conway, W.; Victor, L.; Magilligan, D.; Shiro, F.; Zovick, F.; Roth, T.: Adverse effects of tracheostomy for sleep apnea. J. Am. Med. Ass. *246:* 347–350 (1981).

26   Smith, A.: Courses and classifications of impotence. Urol. Clin. North Am. *8:* 79–90 (1981).

27   Martin, L.: Impotence in diabetes: an overview. Psychosomatics *22:* 318–329 (1981).

28   Furlow, W.: Patient partner satisfaction levels with the inflatable penile prosthesis. J. Am. Med. Ass. *243:* 1714 (1980).

29   Gittes, R.; Waters, W.: Sexual impotence: The overlooked complication of a second renal transplant. J. Urol. *121:* 719 (1979).

30   Van Arsdalen, K.; Klein, F.; Hackler, R.; Brady, S.: Penile implants in spinal cord injury for maintaining external appliances. J. Urol. *126:* 331–332 (1981).

31   Krane, R.; Siroky, M.. Neurophysiology of erection. Urol. Clin. North Am. *8:* 91–102 (1981).

32   Weiss, H.: The physiology of penile erection. Ann. Int. Med. *76:* 793–799 (1972).

33   Spark, R.; White, R.; Connolly, P.: Impotence is not always psychogenic. J. Am. Med. Ass. *243:* 75–755 (1980).

34   Morgan, J.; Pryor, J.: The investigation of organic impotence. Brit. J. Urol. *52:* 571–574 (1980).

35   Lysson, L.; Moore, D.; Pope, A.; Todd, F.; Avilo, S.: Sexual dysfunction in hypertensive diabetic men. J. Cardiovasc. Med.; Special Supplement, April (1981).

36   Casey, W.: Phallography: technique and results of nocturnal tumescence monitoring. J. Urol. *122:* 750–732 (1979).

37   Karacan, I.: Nocturnal penile tumescence as a biological marker in assessing erectile dysfunction. Psychosomatics *23:* 349–360 (1982).

38   Stewart, T.: Sex, spinal cord injury, and staff rapport. Rehabilit. Lit. *42:* 347–350 (1981).

39   Abel, G.; Becker, J.; Cunningham-Rathner, J.; Mittelman, M.; Primack, M.: Differential diagnosis of impotence in diabetics: the validity of sexual symptomatology. Neurol. Urodyn. *1:* 57–59 (1982).

40   Gee, W.; McRoberts, W.; Raney, J.; Amell, J.: The impotent patients: surgical treatment with penile prosthesis and psychiatric evaluation. J. Urol. *111:* 41–43 (1974).

41   Stewart, T.; Gerson, S.: Penile prosthesis: Psychological factors. Urol. *7:* 400–402 (1978).

42   Renshaw, D.: Inflatable penile prosthesis. J. Am. Med. Ass. *241:* 2637–2638 (1979).

43   Kramarsky-Binkhorst, S.: Female perception of Small-Carrion implant. Urol. *12:* 545–548 (1978).

44   Ficher, M.; Zuckerman, M.; Fishkin, P.; Goldman, A.; Neeb, M.; Fink, P.; Cohen, S.; Jacobs, J.; Weisberg, M.: Do endocrines play an etiologic role in diabetic and nondiabetic sexual dysfunctions? ANDROL *5 (1):* 8–16 (1984 Jan.–Feb.).

45   Murray, L.: Sexual dysfunction in diabetics. Sexual Medicine Today. November, pp. 11–15 (1982).

46   Bohannon, M.J.; Zilbergeld, B.; Bulard, D.; Stoklosa, J.: Treatable impotence in diabetic patients. West. J. Med. *136:* 6–10 (1982).

47   Narayana. S.; Loening, S.; Hawtrey, C.; Bonney, W.; Fallon, B.; Gerber, W.; Culp, D.: Penile prosthesis for the treatment of impotence. Brit. J. Urol. *52:* 575–578 (1980).

48   American Medical Systems: Minneapolis Manufacturer of the Scott.

49   Dacomed Corporation. Minneapolis Manufacturer of the Jonas.

50   Gaur, D.: Single implant in the treatment of erectile impotence. J. Urol. *126:* 745–746 (1981).

51   Seagraves, R.; Schoenberg, H.; Zarins, C.: Psychosexual adjustment after penile prosthetic surgery. Manuscript.

52   Smith, A.; Lange, P.; Fraley, E.: A comparison of the Small-Carrion and Scott-Bradley penile prosthesis. J. Urol. *121:* 26–28 (1979).

53   Klein, L.: Personal Communication.

Thomas D. Stewart, MD, Harvard Medical School, Boston, MA 02215 (USA)

Subject Index